APPROACHES
to BEHAVIOR

Changing the dynamic between patients and
professionals in diabetes care and education

Janis Roszler, MS, RD, LD/N, CDE, FAND,
and Wendy Satin Rapaport, PsyD, LCSW

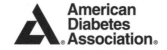

American
Diabetes
Association

Director, Book Publishing, Abe Ogden; *Managing Editor,* Greg Guthrie; *Acquisitions Editor,* Victor Van Beuren; *Production Manager,* Melissa Sprott; *Production Services,* Cenveo Publisher Services; *Cover Design,* Kim Woody; *Printer,* Data Reproductions Corp.

Printed in the United States of America
1 3 5 7 9 10 8 6 4 2

The suggestions and information contained in this publication are generally consistent with the *Clinical Practice Recommendations* and other policies of the American Diabetes Association, but they do not represent the policy or position of the Association or any of its boards or committees. Reasonable steps have been taken to ensure the accuracy of the information presented. However, the American Diabetes Association cannot ensure the safety or efficacy of any product or service described in this publication. Individuals are advised to consult a physician or other appropriate health care professional before undertaking any diet or exercise program or taking any medication referred to in this publication. Professionals must use and apply their own professional judgment, experience, and training and should not rely solely on the information contained in this publication before prescribing any diet, exercise, or medication. The American Diabetes Association—its officers, directors, employees, volunteers, and members—assumes no responsibility or liability for personal or other injury, loss, or damage that may result from the suggestions or information in this publication.

∞ The paper in this publication meets the requirements of the ANSI Standard Z39.48-1992 (permanence of paper).

ADA titles may be purchased for business or promotional use or for special sales. To purchase more than 50 copies of this book at a discount, or for custom editions of this book with your logo, contact the American Diabetes Association at booksales@diabetes.org.

American Diabetes Association
1701 North Beauregard Street
Alexandria, Virginia 22311

DOI: 10.2337/9781580405386

Library of Congress Cataloging-in-Publication Data
Roszler, Janis, author.
 Approaches to behavior : changing the dynamic between patients and professionals in diabetes care and education / Janis Roszler, Wendy Satin Rapaport.
    p. ; cm.
Includes bibliographical references and index.
ISBN 978-1-58040-538-6 (alk. paper)
 I. Rapaport, Wendy Satin, 1947- author. II. American Diabetes Association, issuing body. III. Title.
 [DNLM: 1. Attitude of Health Personnel. 2. Diabetes Mellitus--therapy. 3. Health Communication. 4. Professional-Family Relations. 5. Professional-Patient Relations. WK 815]
 RC660
 616.4'62--dc23
                    2014008450

To the professors who inspired me as a student at UMass Boston's Marriage and Family Therapy program: Drs. Gonzalo Bacigalupe, Alisa Beaver, Esmaeil Mahdavi, MaryAnna Ham, Dawn Shelton, and Margarita Tarragona. Your insightful life lessons transformed how I interact with others. May you continue to inspire your students to learn, grow, and reach out to those in need.

—Janis Roszler

To my wonderful husband Jim, my soul mate and inspiration, who makes me dig deep to be a better wife to a person who has diabetes.

—Wendy Satin Rapaport

Contents

Preface vii

Acknowledgments ix

1 Who's to Blame?. 1
   Everyone plays a role in communication

2 Set the Stage 11
   The environment matters

3 Connecting With Your Patients 31
   Ways to build communication pathways

4 For Your Toolbox, Part I. 47
   Approaches to use with patients

5 For Your Toolbox, Part II 61
   More approaches to use with patients

6 Emotions: Yours, Mine, and Ours 75
   How you and your patients may feel

7 It Takes a Village 89
   Group communication

8 Singing Kumbaya 105
   Workplace communication

9 All in the Family. 117
   Communication with patients and their families

10 Heading Home 131
     Ways to emotionally transition from work to home
     References and Resources. 143
     Index 161

Preface

As a health care professional you have a wealth of knowledge to share. So why don't some of your patients listen, participate, and follow through?

This book examines the emotional "noise" that makes it more difficult for patients to gain from interactions they have with you, their health care provider. Some of the interference comes from the patients themselves. Living with a chronic disease like diabetes can prompt such feelings as worry, anger, fear, guilt, frustration, and denial that make it harder for patients to learn, collaborate, and make behavioral decisions. Some of the "noise" may also come from you—your mood, energy level, frustration, and even patience level can accompany you in the conversations you have with patients. So, as you read, we not only will focus on your patients' feelings and emotions, but also will discuss yours as well.

This book focuses on evidence-supported "strength-based" resiliency strategies from family therapy, cognitive–behavioral therapy, emotionally focused therapy, and positive psychology (Norcross, 2002, Hofmann, 2012, Johnson, 2012, Seear, 2013). Many strategies are based on two assumptions: *1)* We affect our patients and others in our lives in a bidirectional or circular way—how we feel and act affects how others respond and vice versa; and *2)* it is not possible to fully understand another person's life experience; to gain information about another person, one must respectfully ask questions and not make assumptions.

The guidance we share within this book is not only for those who work with patients who have diabetes. It also is for health care providers who work with individuals who have any challenging medical issue. If you are just beginning your training, read through the entire book first and fill its margins with your personal thoughts. Take a careful look at your own behaviors, both in your work setting and outside of it. Many of the approaches we share can help you communicate more effectively with everyone in your life, not only with your patients and their families but also with loved ones, acquaintances, and colleagues, especially in this era of integrated care. Refer to this book often as you move through your program.

If you are a seasoned health care professional, we invite you to read through the entire book as well. Be introspective and explore the different ways to handle strong emotions you may feel, from time to time, that may be prompted by stresses in today's health care environment. Use what we share to help you become an even more effective provider, partner, and friend. Many of the approaches may be new to you. We hope that you find them invigorating and effective. We use them ourselves and know how transformative they can be.

The DAWN2 (Diabetes Attitudes Wishes and Needs) study showed that "support which focuses on both clinical and the psychosocial needs of people with diabetes and their families is necessary to ensure successful treatment outcomes" (Novo Nordisk A/S, 2013). The approaches we present in this book can help achieve that goal and can enable you to bring your best self to every personal encounter, at work, and in other areas of your life.

Acknowledgments

I would like to acknowledge Melissa Brail, LMFT, program director, Jewish Community Services of South Florida, for her sage advice, and Maxine Cohn for her incomparable writing guidance. I also would like to thank Wendy for her thoughtful and enthusiastic collaboration and Victor Van Beuren and the hard-working American Diabetes Association publishing team for giving us this wonderful opportunity.

—Janis Roszler

Thirty five years ago, I was hired by Dr. Jay Skyler at the Diabetes Research Institute, University of Miami Medical School. It was a time when medicine rarely included psychologists and social workers on their teams. He was ahead of his time in recognizing the connection between emotions and diabetes. Today we have made incredible strides in health psychology and now recognize its essential role not just as an adjunct for difficult cases but as a necessary component of work with all patients and their families. From the beginning, I felt I really came to understand the "Person" in diabetes through my dearest friend and collaborator Gary Kleiman. Barbara Singer, Suzanne Wolfson, Maureen Murray, and Ellen Ullman added depth and perspective. I am thankful for the opportunities I have had with my colleagues and patients at the DRI, with Dr. Daniel Mintz at the head, along with Drs. Goldberg, Meninghini, and Nemery.

Thanks to Dr. Sandy Bernstein, Psychologist; Suzanne Pallot, MSW; Marilyn Charwat, psychotherapist; and Carole Weinstein, MA; for keeping me grounded in respect for "psychology's place." And thanks to my sisters, Marcia Lavipour and Mary Ellen Schwab, also professionals, who likewise keep me "alert" (as only siblings can do!).

Thanks to my loving nieces, nephews, and brothers-in-law and to our "kids" Bruce and Teri, Dean and Jen, and our granddaughter Chelsi.

Thanks to my friends for their connection.

And thank you, Janis, for inviting me to join you in writing this book. Your originality and creativity are invigorating.

—Wendy Satin Rapaport

1
Who's to Blame?

It's not you, it's me.... You're giving me the "It's not you, it's me" routine? I invented "It's not you, it's me." Nobody tells me it's them, not me. If it's anybody, it's me.
—George Costanza, *Seinfeld*

In this chapter, you will learn the following:

- The mutual influence you and your patients have on each other
- How to start your day more effectively
- The *stop, drop, and roll* intervention

We're in This Together

Have you ever had a patient break down and cry? As a health care provider, you probably have had more than your share of challenging encounters with patients who come to an appointment or group session with emotions that make it harder for you to provide your best care. Think of the patient who is angry, or the one who aggressively counters everything you say with a quote from a television host or noncredentialed Internet blogger. Who's to blame for these tough interactions? We are willing to bet that many of your colleagues, and perhaps you as well, place the blame squarely on the shoulders of the *difficult* patients. If that's the case, we'd like to invite you to adopt a more enlightened, circular, mutually influencing perspective toward these encounters.

When patients enter a session in a difficult mood, it can make it much harder for them to hear what you have to say and remember the guidance you provide. Their emotional state at the time of your interaction provides one possible answer to that age-old question, "Why didn't my patient do what I said?" But, what part might *your* emotions play in this patient–health care provider tango? Your body language, level of enthusiasm, and focus affects how patients respond to you. It's a circular *relationship*—your mood affects your patient's mood and vice versa. A back and forth occurs between both of you. Once the meeting you have with your first patient brings you down, you are more likely to take that "down feeling" into the session with the next patient and negatively affect that relationship as well.

An Israeli study (Kushnir, 2011) examined the impact physicians' moods had on their patient interactions. On "good-mood days," the subjects verbally interacted with their patients for a significantly longer amount of time, whereas those who entered the exam rooms with a negative attitude not only conversed less with their patients, but also increased the number of prescriptions they wrote and referrals they made. According to Fiscella (2004), patients who receive more positive verbal attention from their health care providers place greater trust in them.

The level of trust patients have in their health care providers forms the "cornerstone" of the patient–health care provider relationship (Weng, 2008). Trust also enhances healing (Mikesell, 2013). Hojat (2011) observed that patients who interacted with caring, empathetic physicians were "significantly more likely" to have better A1C values (56%) than those who interacted with less empathetic doctors (40%, $P < 0.001$). A greater number also enjoyed better low-density lipoprotein cholesterol (LDL-C) control (59%) versus those with less empathetic doctors (44%, $P < 0.001$).

Both you and your patient share responsibility for the quality of interaction that takes place when you meet. You are both part of the system; you affect your patients and they affect you. Sorry, George. It's not you, it's not me . . . it's *us*.

Starting Your Day

How you start your day and how you temper your mood and your thoughts can help achieve more effective and fulfilling interactions for you, your patients, loved ones, colleagues, and friends.

"Peggy," a registered nurse and diabetes educator, barely made it to work on time. After hitting the snooze alarm repeatedly, she finally dragged herself out of bed. She was in no mood to go to work. Then she tried on several outfits, each feeling too tight for the long day she had ahead. As she stormed out the door, she breezed by her husband and ignored his question about their plans for the evening. When she entered the office, without as much as a good morning, her boss (Dr. G) ordered her to meet with Mrs. X, a patient he refused to see; Mrs. X got on his nerves and he wasn't in the mood to meet with her that morning. As Peggy entered the exam room, Mrs. X greeted her by saying, "I don't know how you can help me—you're just as overweight as I am!" That sealed it. What followed was a series of negative "pay it forwards." Peggy started her day off badly with negative thoughts and carried them with her throughout the rest of the day.

How do you start your day? Is it in a hurried and emotional rush or do you make every effort to bring your best self to the important work you do? Do you counter challenges you have throughout the morning with positive self-talk or do you let the "small stuff" negatively affect your mood? Here are a few things you can try to be more focused and emotionally prepared:

Reducing Sleep Inertia

When your alarm goes off in the morning, how do you respond? If you struggle to wake up each morning, you may be suffering from sleep inertia. That is the unpleasant, groggy feeling many people experience immediately after they open their eyes in the morning. Sleep inertia can last as short as 5 minutes or as long as 4 hours, but generally it doesn't last longer than 30 minutes and can make it much harder for you to get going in the morning. The occurrence of sleep inertia has a lot to do with the sleep stage you are in just before waking up. "Abrupt awakening during a slow wave sleep (SWS) episode produces more sleep inertia than awakening in stage 1 or 2, REM sleep being intermediate" (Tassi, 2000).

How can you reduce your sleep inertia or prevent it from occurring? Get more sleep, because sleep deprivation increases the amount of slow wave sleep you have (Tassi, 2000). You also can try using a different type of alarm clock. An "artificial dawn" light alarm system can significantly reduce your level of sleep inertia (Gimenez, 2010). It doesn't rely on the traditional buzz or ring sound to wake you up. Instead, like a natural sunrise, the artificial dawn light gradually becomes brighter and brighter as it gently arouses you. It is a relatively inexpensive item that you set to go on just before your desired wake up time. If you can't get to bed earlier, you may find it helpful to schedule a brief nap during the day to refresh yourself. If your nap is between 5–15 minutes, you can enjoy an immediate energy bump that may last from 1–3 hours. If your nap is longer than 30 minutes, you initially may experience another groggy period of sleep inertia when you wake up, but will eventually go onto enjoy "improved cognitive performance" for quite a few hours (Lovato, 2010).

Managing Negative Messages

Peggy, in our scenario, heeded several negative inner messages that affected her behavior. While getting dressed, her critical inner voice urged her to recall how much she disliked her appearance. When her husband asked about their evening plans, that same voice reminded her that she was still angry at him about a comment he made the night before. That critical inner voice can be a powerful advisor: If you welcome its negative messages, you are more likely to have a tough day. The good news is that you have the ability to convert negative messages into more positive ones.

In 2012, a group of French researchers observed locals in a nearby barroom. They noted that the more alcohol the patrons consumed, the more attractive they believed themselves to be. Next, using a balanced placebo design, the researchers divided 94 subjects into two separate groups; one received alcoholic drinks while the other received nonalcoholic ones. Half of the members of both groups were told that their beverages were alcoholic and the other half were told that their drinks were alcohol free. After everyone finished drinking, all participants were asked to tape a video speech and rate how "attractive, bright, original, and funny" they believed they were. Independent judges who viewed the tapes found that those who believed they had imbibed alcohol awarded themselves more positive ratings. The assumption they made about their drinks affected their inner voices. This study, published in the *British Journal of Psychology*, goes by the following title: Beauty is in the Eye of the "Beer" Holder! (Bègue, 2012).

Stop, Drop, and Roll!

The barroom patrons coincidentally adjusted their inner voice after learning that their beverage contained alcohol. You also can change your inner voice deliberately. To do this, simply stop, drop, and roll (SDR). If you grew up in the United States, your elementary school teacher probably taught you the SDR fire safety technique to use if your clothing or hair ever caught fire. You were told to *1) stop* moving, *2) drop* to the floor and cover your face, and *3) roll* back and forth to extinguish the flames. Here is our version:

1. **Stop.** Stop what you are doing and breathe. Then identify the negative thought you just received from your critical inner voice. (If you find it helpful, visualize a red stop sign.)
2. **Drop.** Drop the negative message about yourself or your patient and adopt a calmer, more generous, and compassionate one.
3. **Roll.** Roll forward with your new approach to the situation. If your feelings are particularly strong, you may need to repeat steps 1 and 2 multiple times before you feel comfortable enough to move forward.

Let's return to our original scenario:

Dr. G had no intention of seeing Mrs. X. Despite his urging, Mrs. X refused to check her fasting blood glucose level every morning and that infuriated him. When he learned that she was coming to see him that morning, he felt angry and frustrated. He thought to himself, "Why doesn't she listen? Why does she ignore the important self-management care tasks I assign?" Dr. G's frustration put him in a horrible mood; he didn't think he could speak with her without becoming angry. So, he told Peggy to see Mrs. X as soon as she arrived.

If Dr. G had used SDR, he might have enjoyed a more satisfying session with Mrs. G. as follows:

1. **Stop.** Dr. G. would recognize that he was angry and frustrated by Mrs. X's behavior. He felt bad because his anger affected his ability to care for her.
2. **Drop.** Dr. G. would drop his negative thoughts and adopt a calmer, more generous, and compassionate understanding of Mrs. X's behavior. Maybe mornings were too hectic for her or she didn't understand why she should test her blood. Maybe she resented having diabetes or felt impatient because her blood glucose level was running high. Maybe knowing that she had a bad morning glucose value made her feel like a failure, so she didn't want to do it. Dropping a negative attitude can be very challenging to do, but it is possible. For many, the key to doing this is to take a moment

and consider the situation from the other person's point of view. No one is all bad or all good. As a healer, take time to tap into your compassionate side and give the other person the benefit of the doubt.

- **Roll.** Dr. G would be ready to move forward. He would immediately calm down and choose to talk to Mrs. X about her reluctance to check her blood in a kinder, more understanding way. They would discuss the issue and come up with a solution: Mrs. X would check her morning blood glucose level twice a week on days when her schedule was less demanding. She also learned how to interpret her results and view them as helpful data, not threatening comments about her behavior.

Use the SDR intervention with patients, family, friends, staff, and even with yourself. It's easy to remember, especially when you feel overwhelmed by strong, emotions. SDR can help you maintain a more positive attitude throughout the day. At the start of this chapter, we invited you to see your interactions with others as being circular—your behavior affects theirs and vice versa. When you use SDR to change your thinking, you bring a new, more positive perspective to each encounter. Your altered attitude can affect their behavior in a different, hopefully more positive, way. Throughout this book, we will show you how to use this tool and share it with your patients to help them better deal with the frustrations of living with diabetes and other challenging medical issues.

What to Eat?

According to the American Diabetes Association (ADA), "current evidence does not strongly support one eating pattern (such as Mediterranean, vegetarian, or low carbohydrate) over another" for managing diabetes in adults (ADA, 2013). That said, how you eat can affect your mood. A team at the University of Navarra followed the relationship between food choices and depression in 10,094 healthy individuals without depression. They found, after 4.4 years, that subjects who adhered more strictly to a Mediterranean diet were 42% less likely to develop depression.

In the study, the Mediterranean diet was defined as a "high ratio of mono-unsaturated fats (i.e., olive oil) to saturated fats; moderate intake of alcohol and dairy products; low intake of meat; and high intake of legumes, fruit and nuts, cereals, vegetables and fish." (Sánchez-Villegas, 2009). Those who consumed larger amounts of dairy and meat products increased their risk of depression significantly (Sánchez-Villegas, 2009). Proponents of this way of eating also encourage people to be physically active, get adequate rest, and join others for food preparation and meals.

In other words, "all work and no play" doesn't bode well for a healthy life. Regardless of how you choose your foods, people who feel more upbeat and energized are more likely to enjoy meaningful interactions.

The Commute (Ugh!) and How to Transition to a Better Day

Now it's time to head to work. You are well-rested, well-fed, energized, and ready to connect with your patients. Then, you hit traffic. How do you respond to honking cars, rude drivers, and slow-moving traffic? Do you feel your blood come to a boil or do you stay calm? If it unnerves you, how well do you calm yourself once you enter your office? You can choose to see traffic from a more positive point of view. Think of it as an unexpected, but welcome, break in your hectic day. It is private time when you can listen to music or to a favorite talk show. Don't take calls, but answer the phone quickly and say you will call back when you arrive at work. If you view these extra minutes as free time, the delay is less likely to frustrate you. Just let co-workers know you are caught in traffic so they can make any necessary scheduling adjustments. Then try to enjoy that private time.

I *Like* Traffic

I am lucky
I am free
I get extra time
with only me

and if I think
that I am boring
I use audible.com
to go exploring

I say this
when I begin my drive
I will arrive happy
. . . and *alive*

—Dr. Wendy Satin Rapaport

Calming Tools
Physical Activity

Many of us turn to physical activity to help reduce our stress: We do yoga, work out at the gym, or fit in a brisk 10-minute walk to help handle the tensions of the day. The following are additional calming techniques you can try. Your personal experience with these can help you communicate their value to others.

Deep Breathing

Breathing comes naturally, but the types of breaths we take when we are tense tend to be more shallow and quick. Joan Borysenko, director of Harvard's Mind-Body Program, suggests diaphragmatic breathing as a way to calm yourself when you are stressed (Borysenko, 2011). To breathe this way, do the following:

- Take a slow, deep breath as you expand your belly then exhale slowly. This will help you calm down. To take this breathing to the next level, assess the amount of stress you currently feel and assign it a number from 1 to 10, with 10 being the most anxious. Next, take that number of deep, slow, diaphragmatic breaths and gradually feel yourself move from your high stress number to a much lower, calmer number.
- Focus on your belly as you inhale. Hold the breath for a few moments then slowly exhale as you watch your belly contract. Inhale, hold, exhale, repeat . . . silently recite these steps, if you find it helpful. Try to remember how it feels to calm yourself down from a high stress level to a calmer level. If thoughts enter your mind, let them pass without judgment and return your focus back to your breathing.
- Enjoy the increased level of calm that you start to feel.

Breathing on the Go

When you don't have time to run through a complete breathing exercise or are at locations where deep breathing isn't practical, such as in a meeting, focus on a time when you did the exercise and picture the tension flowing out of your body. Your recollection of this activity can calm you down, even if you don't run through an entire breathing sequence. If possible, close your eyes for a moment and feel your body move from a high level of stress to a calmer level.

Mindfulness

Mindfulness is all about training your brain to slow down and "smell the roses." Life is hectic. We juggle overwhelming schedules and multitask. When you practice mindfulness, you focus only on the present. As thoughts and feelings enter your mind, don't judge them, as they are neither good nor bad. Just breathe and stay in the moment. This is a great technique to use when life becomes chaotic.

Minute Visualization

Stop what you are doing, breathe, and take a moment to return to a calming memory, feeling, or place. If nothing comes to mind, think about something you enjoy in nature. The added visualization can help reinforce a deeper feeling of relaxation. As you breathe, repeat a phrase that makes you smile or relax, such as "children laughing" or "the smell of coffee in the morning," and see what happens.

Guided Imagery Meditation

Choose a phrase that has meaning for you then focus on it as you take five slow, deep breaths. One example is the phrase "the joy of helping." As you repeat it, remember the warm feeling of satisfaction that radiates throughout your body as you experience the joy of helping others. Breathe in, and out—*the joy of helping, the joy of helping*—as you say the words, feel happy about the work you do. If you work with children, feel the warmth of a tiny hand clutching your hand as you help bring comfort to a young one newly diagnosed with diabetes. *The joy of helping*—picture the slight nodding of the father's head as he holds back tears. Your eyes meet and connect. You give him hope. *The joy of helping*—picture the 50-year-old woman shocked by her diagnosis, but who no longer feels alone because she is with you. *The joy of helping... the joy of helping.* Remember these powerful images and keep the memories with you throughout the day.

Remember, you have some control over your day. Use the SDR intervention and the other techniques we mentioned to help change your thinking. Try to calm yourself before you enter your workplace. The minutes you invest in doing this may improve your physical and mental health, as well as the interactions you have with your staff, patients, and other people you encounter throughout the day. So, check your bad mood at the door, leave it in the car, or make an effort to moderate it as your day goes on. It's good for you *and* your patients.

The Takeaway

Be mindful of how you, your health, and your emotions affect others.

2
Set the Stage

In this chapter, you will learn the following:

- How to promote better patient and professional interactions *before* you meet

Have you ever seen the Ellen DeGeneres show? She has one of the most enthusiastic audiences on television. When Ellen walks out onto the stage at the start of the show, the crowd goes wild. Within minutes everyone is cheering and dancing in the aisles. How do the individual audience members, who certainly look forward to seeing the host, transform into a supercharged group? Ellen's staff gets a lot of the credit; they greet each visitor with lots of enthusiasm, play lively music, dance, and joke around with everyone. Because they put in such an effort *before* the curtain goes up, Ellen gets a great response from the crowd and has a terrific show.

Who "warms up" your patients before they meet with you? Your staff. They schedule appointments and greet everyone who comes to see you. How well does your staff interact with your patients? Are they caring and attentive or rude, hostile, or indifferent? Don't underestimate their role as your personal ambassadors. We know many patients who've dropped health care providers because they disliked the way they were treated by the office staff. Like you, your support staff must be able to handle difficult patients-related situations with aplomb and behave in professional ways, that is, they should never complain or argue with one another within the earshot of your patients.

Transforming Your Waiting Area

Does your waiting area communicate your healing perspective? Step into your office and look at it through your patients' eyes. What are they likely to see, hear, and feel as they enter? Does the environment reduce stress or heighten it?

Dr. Francesca Gallarello, a Miami Beach cardiologist, transformed the small, dingy waiting area of her new office into a serene outdoor setting. She brought in sleek, white couches, a live plant arrangement, and papered the largest wall with a life-size photo of a European street scene. As patients wait, they are calmed by this soothing environment. Your office space should be clean, attractive, engaging, and relaxing. The furniture should not be worn or broken and, yes, your magazines should be current. If possible, display some form of nature, be it natural or artificial. A group of Dutch researchers examined the stress-lowering effects of real and artificial plants in a hospital waiting room. They found that "adding real or artificial natural elements to health care environments provides an unobtrusive and inexpensive stress and anxiety management method" (Beukeboom, 2012).

Take the "Wait" Out of the Waiting Area

With today's time constraints, most patients are likely to spend a significant amount of time in waiting rooms. Unfortunately, longer wait times are associated with reduced patient satisfaction (Anderson, 2007). Those who must wait a long time to see you are more likely to be upset, impatient, and angry by the time you finally do meet. It is certainly appropriate to thank them for their patience, but because lengthy waits are often unavoidable, try to use the time to educate your patients and help them prepare to meet with you.

One way to utilize the wait time is to physically prepare your patients to be as alert as possible when they interact with you. If you work with individuals who have diabetes, check their blood glucose level as soon as they arrive. Most offices check glucose levels after patients get assigned to an exam room. Shortly after that, you, their health care provider, usually will enter the room. If a patient has a low glucose level, he or she won't have adequate time to improve it before seeing you, so you may end up interacting with someone who can't give you undivided attention. Some of your messages will reach their intended target, whereas others may be missed entirely. If your patients get their blood checked when they sign in, they should have adequate time to respond to a snack or take a corrective dose of insulin, if needed. If they don't have a snack handy, provide one along with a handout on how to treat hypoglycemia. By the time the two of you meet, your patient's glucose level should be within, or at least closer to a desired target range, which should help you both communicate more effectively.

Educate

Transform your waiting room into an extension of your treatment. Many health care providers do this. They display informative brochures, hang posters, and even mount televisions that run educational programming (Gignon, 2012). These are helpful tools that add value to the waiting room experience. But, they are passive activities. For more active learning, invite your patients to complete worksheets that heighten their self-awareness, challenge negative beliefs, help them identify strengths, and utilize their problem-solving skills. Near the worksheets, post the following: "Your appointment starts now. Please fill out these forms."

Setting the Agenda

We designed the following worksheets for you to use in your waiting area. They contain thought-provoking questions that can help your patients consider their medically related psychological, social, and behavioral issues in a more positive and proactive way. These sheets aren't just busy work. Writing about stressful experiences and health-related issues can speed up healing (Smyth, 1999). Expressive writing also helps many individuals enjoy improvements in their mood, emotional and physical symptoms, and immune system functioning (Baikie, 2005). If desired, use these worksheets to set the agenda for the appointment. If you don't want to use them in that way, try to acknowledge your patients' effort. Patients want you to take an interest in what they've accomplished or learned. Your inquiry doesn't have to take up a lot of time. Simply ask your patients to name one or two things they gained from doing this activity.

Some of these worksheets are diabetes focused and are based on the American Association of Diabetes Educators' list (the AADE7™) of seven self-care behaviors: healthy eating, being active, monitoring, taking medications, problem solving, healthy coping, and reducing risks. Several worksheets cover generic health-related issues. If you deal with a different area of medicine or have other topics you would like to address, create worksheets of your own. For example, you can develop worksheets on intimacy, humor, body image, relapse challenges, and motivation. Use simple, clear language to accommodate patients with reading difficulties and be sure to include questions that help your patients access their problem-solving strengths.

Worksheet Theme Guide

Worksheet 1. Value of Support
Worksheet 2. Personal Beliefs
Worksheet 3. Power of Positive Thinking
Worksheet 4. Setting Personal Goals
Worksheet 5. Being Thankful
Worksheet 6. Dealing With Stress
Worksheet 7. Eating Healthy
Worksheet 8. Being Active
Worksheet 9. Monitoring Blood Glucose
Worksheet 10. Feeling Overwhelmed or Frustrated
Worksheet 11. Learning New Skills
Worksheet 12. Understanding the Positive Power of the Diabetes Police

Worksheet 1. Value of Support

Did you know that . . . **when friends, family, and others support you and your medical issues, they become healthier too?**

Please respond to the questions below. Write on the back, if you need more space.

- In the past, what type of support did you get from friends and loved ones for your medical issues? How did this support make you feel?

- Would you like to have more support now? If so, what type of support do you need?

- How can you ask others to give it to you?

What is one thing you learned from this worksheet that you can share with your health care provider?

Source: Schwartz C, Meisenhelder JB, Ma Y, Reed G: Altruistic social interest behaviors are associated with better mental health. *Psychosom Med* 2003 Sep-Oct;65(5):778–785.

Worksheet 2. Personal Beliefs

Did you know that . . . **what you know, think and believe may help you feel better about your medical issues?**

Please respond to the questions below. Write on the back, if you need more space.

- Why do you think you developed your current medical issue?

- Do you have a belief or view of the world that comforts you? How does this belief affect how you take care of your health?

- How can you use your belief to help you take better care of your health?

What is one thing you learned from this worksheet that you can share with your health care provider?

Source: Jantos M, Kiat H: Prayer as medicine: how much have we learned? *Med J Aust* 2007;186(10 Suppl):S51–S53.

Worksheet 3. Power of Positive Thinking

Did you know that . . . **positive thinking can help you live longer, reduce depression, and overcome many stressful problems?**

Please respond to the questions below. Write on the back, if you need more space.

• What do people admire most about you?

• What do you like best about yourself?

• How can you use these qualities to take better care of your health?

What is one thing you learned from this worksheet that you can share with your health care provider?

Source: Mayo Clinic: Positive thinking: reduce stress by eliminating negative self-talk, n.d. Available at http://www.mayoclinic.com/health/positive-thinking/ SR00009. Accessed 12 July 2013.

Worksheet 4. Setting Personal Goals

Did you know that . . . **you are more likely to become healthier when you set personal goals and take small steps to meet them?**

Please respond to the questions below. Write on the back, if you need more space.

- What health goals would you like to achieve? Take one of your goals and break it into small steps.

- What might get in the way of reaching each of these steps?

- How can you overcome these possible problems?

- Set a deadline for each step and begin your plan!

What is one thing you learned from this worksheet that you can share with your health care provider?

Source: Powers MA: Diabetes BASICS: education, innovation, revolution. *Diabetes Spectr* 19(2):90–98, 2006.

Worksheet 5. Being Thankful

Did you know that . . . **being thankful can help you become healthier?**

Please respond to the questions below. Write on the back, if you need more space.

Many people find that their medical issues improve their lives in some way. They may take better care of their health, are more thankful, or even feel grateful for the things in their lives that are going well.

- What are you thankful for? How can you use these things to motivate you to take actions that help you stay healthy?

- What positive effect have your medical issues had on your life?

- How thankful are you for these changes?

- How have your medical issues positively affected the people around you?

What is one thing you learned from this worksheet that you can share with your health care provider?

Source: Tierney JA: Serving of gratitude may save the day. *New York Times,* page D1, 2011.

Worksheet 6. Dealing With Stress

Did you know that . . . **listening to music can reduce your stress level**?

Please respond to the questions below. Write on the back, if you need more space.

- Doing enjoyable activities can help you relax and improve your health. What types of activities do you enjoy?

- How can you make more time to do the things you enjoy?

- Who can help support your effort to find more time to relax?

- How can you ask them to help you?

What is one thing you learned from this worksheet that you can share with your health care provider?

Source: Mandel SE et al.: Effects of music therapy and music-assisted relaxation and imagery on health-related outcomes in diabetes education a feasibility study. *Diabetes Educ* 39(4):568–581, 2013.

Worksheet 7. Eating Healthy

Did you know that . . . **the food choices you make can help you manage your diabetes and slow or even prevent many complications?**

Please respond to the questions below. Write on the back, if you need more space.

- What healthy food choices do you make?

- How do you feel about making these choices? How can you choose healthy foods more often?

- How can you invite your loved ones to support your need to eat healthier? How can you help them eat healthier also?

What is one thing you learned from this worksheet that you can share with your health care provider?

Source: American Diabetes Association: Nutrition recommendations and interventions for diabetes. *Diabetes Care* 2008;31:S61–S78.

Worksheet 8. Being Active

Did you know that . . . **people who move more, manage their diabetes better, have less stress, and have a lower risk of heart problems?**

Please respond to the questions below. Write on the back, if you need more space.

- Do you do any regular physical activity? What do you do? What part(s) of your workout do you enjoy?

- If you were active, but stopped, what motivated you to be active in the past? How can you use that to help you start moving again?

- If you are active now, how can you maintain or increase your activity level?

- How can you ask others to support your need to be more active (and, maybe help them become more active too)?

What is one thing you learned from this worksheet that you can share with your health care provider?

Source: American Association of Diabetes Educators: Diabetes and physical activity. *Diabetes Educ* 2012;38(1):129–132.

Worksheet 9. Monitoring Blood Glucose

Did you know that . . . **checking your blood glucose level can help you manage your diabetes better?**

Please respond to the questions below. Write on the back, if you need more space.

- How do you feel when you see your blood glucose result on your glucose monitor? How do you feel when the result is not what you expect it to be?

- How can you use these feelings (good or bad) to motivate you to take better care of your health?

- Some people view their glucose monitor as "hiker's compass" that helps keep them on the right track. How do you view your monitor and why?

- How can you use your attitude toward your glucose monitor to help you take better care of your diabetes?

What is one thing you learned from this worksheet that you can share with your health care provider?

Source: Goldstein DE, et al.: Tests of glycemia in diabetes. *Diabetes Care* 27(7):1761–1773, 2004.

Worksheet 10. Feeling Overwhelmed or Frustrated

Did you know that . . . **many people with diabetes feel overwhelmed and frustrated?** Please respond to the questions below. Write on the back, if you need more space.

- Do you ever feel overwhelmed and frustrated with your diabetes? What do you think causes these feelings?

- You have control over how you respond. When you feel that way, what do you do to feel better?

- What type of support can help you feel more upbeat about living with diabetes?

- What steps can you take to get this support?

What is one thing you learned from this worksheet that you can share with your health care provider?

Source: Polonsky WH: Emotional and quality-of-life aspects of diabetes management. *Curr Diab Rep* 2(2):153–159, 2002.

Worksheet 11. Learning New Skills

Did you know that . . . **you may need to learn some new skills to care for your diabetes?**

Please respond to the questions below. Write on the back, if you need more space.

- Diabetes care requires many skills. Some may be easy to learn and some may be harder for you to master. What diabetes skills have you learned to do?

- How do you feel about yourself and all that you have learned?

- How can you use these feelings to motivate yourself to take even better care of your health?

What is one thing you learned from this worksheet that you can share with your health care provider?

Source: American Association of Diabetes Educators. AADE7™. Available at http://www.diabeteseducator.org/ProfessionalResources/AADE7. Accessed 22 May 2014.

Worksheet 12. Understanding the Positive Power of the Diabetes Police

Did you know that . . . **people who nag you about your diabetes care often are called the "Diabetes Police"?**

Please respond to the questions below. Write on the back, if you need more space.

- Do your friends or family ever bother you about your diabetes care? What type of comments do they make to you?

- What do you think motivates them to say these things? Put yourself in their shoes for a moment and consider their point of view. Does this change how you feel about them?

- How do you handle their comments? Do you ever think of their comments as signs that they care about you? Have you ever thanked them for the things they do that help you?

- What have you learned from what they say to you? How can you use their comments to motivate you?

What is one thing you learned from this worksheet that you can share with your health care provider?

Source: Roszler J, et al.: *The Secrets of Living and Loving with Diabetes.* Chicago, IL, Surrey Books, 2004.

These worksheets, hopefully, will encourage your patients to be more thoughtful about their lives and how their behaviors affect their health. After completing a worksheet, your patients may wish to ask you additional questions. As you answer their questions, be sure to acknowledge and praise your patients' interest in caring for their health. If they seem interested, encourage them to suggest worksheet topics that can help them and other patients learn and grow. If they didn't fill out the worksheet, that information is helpful, too. Try to learn and understand why they rejected the assignment.

Recognizing Progress

Our Diabetes Progress Scale is an outgrowth of the strength-based, proactive approach we are promoting throughout this book. We hope that this scale will help patients recognize and appreciate the progress and improvements they have made or hope to make. Living with diabetes or any chronic illness is difficult. Each day is filled with many challenges that many of our patients face with great skill and courage. These efforts deserve recognition. Present this scale in its entirety or choose specific items you wish to share, and give them to your patients while they sit in the waiting room.

The Diabetes Progress Scale

It is not easy to live with diabetes. Think about how far you have come since the day you learned you had diabetes. Read through the following list. Circle the number that shows how impressed you are with how well you do that item. Place a star next to the ones you would like to start doing so you can focus your efforts. Your number rating is not a grade, but rather it is a way for you to increase your awareness of the things you do well.

Scale: 1 = not at all; 2 = a little; 3 = somewhat; 4 = a lot

1. **I'm impressed that . . .** I take care of my diabetes and still want to do my job, enjoy my family and have fun. 1 2 3 4 (*Find balance*)
2. **I'm impressed that . . .** I try not to worry about future problems and focus on living well with diabetes day by day. 1 2 3 4 (*Think positive!*)
3. **I'm impressed that . . .** I ask questions if my health care team wants me to do something I don't understand. 1 2 3 4 (*Search for answers*)
4. **I'm impressed that . . .** I see my blood glucose test results as "feedback," not as negative judgment. 1 2 3 4 (*I don't have to be perfect!*)
5. **I'm impressed that . . .** I know how to ask loved ones for help with some of my diabetes tasks, and do so, when I want it. 1 2 3 4 (*Family support*)
6. **I'm impressed that . . .** I try to follow my meal plan and notice *triggers* that cause me to make poor food choices. 1 2 3 4 (*I'm aware*)
7. **I'm impressed that . . .** When loved ones nag me about my diabetes, I thank them for caring and try to accept their messages in a positive way. 1 2 3 4 (*Think positive!*)
8. **I'm impressed that . . .** I plan ahead, so I can be more active (i.e., I put my sneakers in my car, I make workout plans with others, etc.). 1 2 3 4 (*Create new habits*)
9. **I'm impressed that . . .** I use all the members of my health care team (dentist, eye doctor, dietitian, nurse, psychologist, teachers, etc.) to help me stay healthy. 1 2 3 4 (*I take care of my needs*)
10. **I'm impressed that . . .** If my doctor seems displeased with my progress, I try to hear the care and concern beneath the comments that he or she makes. 1 2 3 4 (*See the good in others*)

11. **I'm impressed that . . .** When I feel like I'm not taking care of my diabetes well, I think of all the health tasks I do well and don't allow my negative feelings to last long. 1 2 3 4 (*Look on the bright side*)

12. **I'm impressed that . . .** I don't let diabetes limit my social life; when I feel good about myself, people respond to my positive attitude. 1 2 3 4 (*I'm important*)

13. **I'm impressed that . . .** When I worry about long-term complications, I remind myself that the better I take care of myself, the healthier I will be. 1 2 3 4 (*Take care of myself*)

14. **I'm impressed that . . .** I can ask my health care team to understand what it's like *for me* to have diabetes. 1 2 3 4 (*I accept myself*)

15. **I'm impressed that . . .** When I feel overwhelmed, I check to see if I feel this way because my blood glucose is out of range or has been swinging high and low. 1 2 3 4 (*I monitor myself*)

16. **I'm impressed that . . .** When I feel overwhelmed, I ask my team to help me set smaller goals. 1 2 3 4 (*Goal setting*)

17. **I'm impressed that . . .** I can help loved ones learn how to support me by talking to them or by bringing them with me to my appointments. 1 2 3 4 (*Build a support team*)

18. **I'm impressed that . . .** What I do also helps educate my loved ones so they can become healthier. 1 2 3 4 (*I'm a good role model!*)

The Takeaway

Set the stage for growth before you meet with your patients.

3
Connecting With Your Patients

Two monologues do not make a dialogue.
—Jeff Daly

In this chapter, you will learn the following:

- How to communicate more effectively with patients who appear emotional, distracted, or unreachable
- How to interact with patients you may not like
- When to refer your patient to a therapist

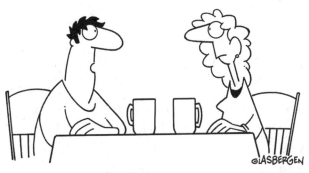

"I'm trying to be a good listener, but you keep breaking my concentration by talking!"

Connecting

Armed with the tools from Chapter one, you hopefully feel more prepared to start your day with a positive mind-set. Even if you enter your office whistling a happy tune, you still are likely to encounter patients who bring their own emotional baggage to their appointments. They may feel angry, sad, frustrated, hopeless, anxious, depressed, hurt, or even guilty about having diabetes or other medical issues. These feelings can be overwhelming, but they are normal. Anticipate them. After all, living with diabetes requires patients to adjust not only their lives but also many of their hopes and dreams. That, alone, can be highly distressing.

You may wish that your patients left these negative feelings at home; however, the fact that they show their emotions so openly may demonstrate how overwhelmed they are feeling as well as how much they trust you and believe you can help them. If you don't acknowledge their feelings in some meaningful way, these emotions can become the proverbial "elephant in the room" and negatively affect everything that happens during your session together. Angry patients, for example, are so distracted by their clenched jaws and throbbing foreheads that they miss many of the important things you say. Your patients' emotions and inability to listen also can affect your mood and prompt you to speak in a more harsh or inappropriate manner.

When Patients Arrive

When you meet with your patients, hand them a sheet of paper on which they can take notes. Think of this handout as their personal prescription pad. On it, they can jot down information you share and suggestions you make, and then they can choose to implement the plans you collaboratively develop more effectively. At the end of the session, ask them to summarize all they learned and tell you what they have decided to do differently before their next visit.

When They Arrive in a Difficult Mood

If you suspect that a patient is not in a positive mood, remember the stop, drop, and roll (SDR) intervention. *Stop* for a moment. *Drop* any negative judgment you have about seeing this person, and *roll* forward with a more compassionate stance before you step into the room. Once you enter the room, set the stage for a meaningful interaction. Think LEAP and follow these four steps:

1. Listen
2. Empathize
3. Affirm
4. Positively reframe

Step 1. Listen

Carl Rogers, the father of client-centered therapy, said the following about the value of being heard:

> I can testify that when you are in psychological distress and someone really hears you without passing judgment on you, without trying to take responsibility for you, without trying to mold you, it feels damn good! (Rogers, 1980)

When you encounter distressed patients, listen carefully to their concerns. Ask open-ended questions to help find out what is really on their minds. If your time is limited, ask them to take a moment and state how they feel in a single word or sentence. That request will help your patients clarify their thoughts and get right to the point. When possible, invite them to share what they have accomplished so far, to remind them of their progress as they consider their struggles. Use body language to demonstrate your sincerity—lean forward, face your patient, and make eye contact. Fight the temptation to glance at your electronic notepad or other devices. We know that should be obvious, but it is a common patient complaint that deserves note (Gualtieri, 2010). Your goal is to feel and communicate genuineness, authenticity, sincerity, and compassion; none of which can be achieved if your attention is elsewhere. Don't worry if you don't know what to say or how to respond. *The fact that you care enough to listen is healing*; it shows your patients that you see them as individuals and want to know how they think and feel. Additionally, when you attend to your patients in this way, they observe how quality listening is done and, hopefully, will employ this behavior in their own lives with emotionally distressed loved ones.

Active listening isn't just a matter of courtesy. There are real rewards for reaching out to others in this way. When you give your patients permission to express how they feel about their diabetes or other distressing concerns, they are more likely to share additional information with you, take their medication as prescribed, show up to follow-up appointments, and follow through with the lifestyle changes you recommend (Bayne, 2013). When you identify a problematic issue, you take the first step toward resolving it. If you aren't convinced yet, consider your wallet as well as your peace of mind. One study showed that physicians who develop empathic relationships with their patients have a lower incidence of malpractice claims (Levasseur, 1993, as cited in Bayne, 2013). This may apply to educators and other professionals as well.

Step 2. Empathize

To reflect a statement your patient shares, repeat it back to him or her in your own words. You can do this compassionately or empathically. What's the difference?

- **Being compassionate:** You feel sympathetic about someone's situation, but you don't try to understand how they feel or explore how deeply they are suffering. For example: Habitat for Humanity helps people in need, so you write a check to the organization and send it off in the mail. You don't read the profiles on the website or try to learn more about the recipients of your gift. You give, because you know the organization is effective and helpful.
- **Being empathic:** You donate to Habitat for Humanity, but you go beyond writing a check. You make an effort to learn about the recipients of your gift— who they are, what matters to them, and how they feel about their current situation. According to Danielle Ofri, author of *What Doctors Feel* (2013a), "this is where doctors often stumble—empathy requires being able to communicate all of this to the patient."

Consider the following compassionate exchange between Mike and his dietitian, Susan:

Mike: Susan, I want to follow my meal plan, but my schedule is too hectic.

Susan: It's not easy to fit diabetes into your busy life. It sounds like you want to follow it, but haven't figured out how to fit it into your life. Is that right? (*Reflect/confirm.*) Let's see what you are willing to do.

Compare that exchange with this empathic exchange:

Mike: Susan, I want to follow my meal plan, but my schedule is too hectic.

Susan: It sounds like you might be upset because you're too busy to follow the meal plan we created last time. Is that right? (*Reflect/confirm.*)

Mike: Yes, I really want to eat well, but my schedule is crazy.

Susan: That must be frustrating, because I know you care a lot about your diabetes. I'd really like to hear about what's getting in your way. (*Empathy.*)

Both being compassionate and empathic are important options that require good listening skills. Being empathic, the gold standard in connecting, takes a little additional time and effort that we believe is well spent. But being compassionate is valuable too. If you don't have time to be empathic with each of your patients, be compassionate.

Step 3. Affirm

The way our patients feel and act is common; they are not alone. Assure Mike that his feelings, even uncomfortable ones, are natural feelings that many people have and will most likely pass:

Susan: Hi, Mike. You're too busy to follow the meal plan we created last time? Thanks for letting me know. That must be aggravating, because you told me how much you care about your health. Many of my patients find that following a new meal plan gets easier with time. (*Affirm.*) Your frustration should decrease as you become more familiar with your plan and start to get into a new routine. It's not easy, but it's worth it.

People respond more positively when they know that others behave the same way they do. In 2010, Dr. Nat Strand became the first individual with type 1 diabetes to win television's *The Amazing Race*, an intensely demanding, global scavenger hunt. Over the course of 23 grueling days, she and her teammate, Dr. Kat Chang, traveled 32,000 miles across four continents, 10 countries, and 31 cities. They raced dog sleds in the Arctic Circle, speed skated in South Korea, and even got lost for a frustrating 6 hours while driving through the deserts of Oman. Their ultimate goal? To win the $1 million prize. Throughout the competition, Nat struggled to keep her blood glucose well-controlled, which dipped into the low 40s and soared into the high 300s when the race became particularly stressful—like the time when she battled her intense fear of heights to leap off a 150-foot crane that hovered over California's Long Beach Pier. Although her experience was far from typical, viewers with diabetes empathized with her efforts to maintain control of her diabetes. After the competition, she received hundreds of supportive messages from folks who were happy to see that, like them, Nat also struggled with abnormal glucose levels (*affirmation*).

Step 4. Positively Reframe

During your session, Mike complains that his wife meddles too much in his diabetes care. She questions his food choices and reminds him to check his blood, even though he doesn't need reminding. He says that she acts this way because she likes to annoy him. You ask if he thinks it is possible that she may do these actions because she cares so deeply about him and his health. The new more optimistic "spin" you offered is a positive reframe. You encourage Mike to thank his wife for caring about him and assure her that she doesn't have to monitor him so closely. If her actions continue to bother him, the couple can meet with the therapist on your team who can help them communicate more effectively with one another.

If the above supportive exchanges aren't your approach, what comes out of your mouth may feel awkward or phony. This is partly because it is new for you; learning to ride a bike or play tennis is also awkward in the beginning. The more you engage in this type of interaction, the more easily you will find wording that fits your personal style and point of view. Even Carl Rogers, quoted earlier, struggled to become adept as a listener (Rogers, 1980). If you want, you can use the "fake it 'till you make it" approach. The truth is that you don't have to *feel* empathic to *act* empathic. As a matter of fact, the more heartfelt comments you make to those around you, the more empathic you are likely to become (Wise, 2013). The good news is that your efforts are not one directional. When you help patients see an issue in a more positive light (positive reframe) that optimistic message also can positively affect how *you* perceive the issue. Try this technique with your family, friends, and others you deal with each day. Observe how it affects your attitude. As you read through this book, we will share additional ways to apply this.

If you think showing empathy compromises your ability to be seen as an expert or crosses some sort of professional boundary, you are mistaken. It increases your competency. When you connect to your patients as individuals and recognize their feelings, you give them permission to have empathy for themselves. Your professional behavior demonstrates how people can take a momentary break from their troubling issues, yet still be aware and responsible. As they follow your lead, they, hopefully, will give themselves emotional breaks as well. When they do, great changes can happen.

After you respond to your patients' initial comments, ask what they'd like to do to take better care of their health. Here is an example: Joan says she feels depressed because the neuropathic pain in her feet forced her to drop out of her favorite aerobics class. This class was an important social outlet for her, which had a positive impact on her mood. Now that it is gone, she fears that she may lose even more parts of her life as her diabetes progresses. How would you respond?

Consider the following possible response:

Tell Joan that you are impressed that, as depressed as she feels, she is still able to recognize how dropping out of this class affects her mood, her diabetes, and her social situation. Next, ask her what she thinks she could to do to meet her physical and social needs. Let her know that therapy can help her manage her fear and keep her negative feelings from affecting her ability to care for her health. If a therapist is not readily available, urge her to participate in a local support group, meet with a spiritual advisor, or reach out to another member of her personal support system. If you are available, you also can offer to set up an additional appointment with her so that the two of you can discuss more of her concerns.

Team Up

Be collaborative and invite your patients to share behavioral changes they feel ready to try. If you want them to become more active, for example, ask what type of physical activity they'd like to do, with whom, and at what time. When you tell people what to do, you assume that you know what is best for their lives. If you urge them to do what you think is best, you initially may get positive results, but you also may undermine their confidence and ability to come up with future self-care strategies of their own. Inviting them to brainstorm with you helps them develop healthy problem-solving behaviors when you are not around (Berg, 2012).

If you have a secure work e-mail, share it with your patients and invite them to tell you about positive moments they encounter between appointments. According to the U.S. Department of Health and Human Services, HIPAA's Privacy Rule "allows covered health care providers to communicate electronically, such as through e-mail, with their patients, provided they apply reasonable safeguards when doing so" (Health Information Privacy, 2008). It is not necessary to send a lengthy response. Just tell them to expect to hear back from you and then reply with a happy face ":)" or a simple "Great!" to let them know you received and enjoyed their message.

Positive e-mail interactions and other innovative communication options help support your patients and reinforce important health messages while you are apart.

Explore Cultural Beliefs

To help you learn more about your patients' cultural views about diabetes, ask the following three questions (Anderson, 2002):

- What does having diabetes mean to you?
- What does having diabetes mean in your family?
- What does having diabetes mean in your community?

Then work with your patients and their family members with areas of concern.

In some ethnic communities, "a diabetes diagnosis reflects a personal failure of consuming excess calories, behaving immorally, or being unspiritual" (Anderson, 2002). A wife of a Latino man, for example, may blame herself for causing her husband's diabetes, if she is the one who is responsible for food preparation in the family (Anderson, 2002). Ask about family, holiday, or religious customs that affect how your patients care for their diabetes. If they participate in the month-long practice of fasting until sundown to mark the holiday of Ramadan, you may need to help them adjust their insulin dose, so they don't experience fasting-related hypoglycemia or hyperglycemia (Anderson, 2002). For assistance with Ramadan, we suggest *Recommendations for Management of Diabetes During Ramadan* (Al-Arouj, 2009).

If your patients are of the Jewish faith and want to follow the Passover holiday's dietary restrictions, help them locate dietary information that helps them consume appropriate portions of the foods commonly eaten on that holiday, such as products prepared with matzo. One website that offers helpful diabetes-related Passover information is http://www.Friendswithdiabetes.com.

Lessons That Linger

Here is how the supportive interactions you have with your patients can positively influence their behaviors in the future:

Ted stopped at a nearby coffee shop to pick up a decaf coffee. While waiting in line, he spied a croissant that had his name written all over it. In the past, he would have impulsively added it to his order, gobbled it down, and then hated himself for the rest of the day regardless of how well he ate later. But this time was different. At a recent appointment, his diabetes educator, Samantha, recognized how frustrated he was about his eating urges and reminded him that he tended to feel that way when his blood glucose level ran high. They brainstormed and Ted identified several ideas he thought he might like to try:

- He could go to a different coffee shop and develop a new, croissant-free, coffee-purchasing tradition.
- He could bring exact change for the coffee, so he wouldn't purchase anything else.
- He should give himself permission to stop feeling guilty because he wants to eat the croissant. Having diabetes doesn't mean he has to deny himself everything he loves.
- He could use pre- and post-blood glucose checks to see how the croissant affects his efforts to manage his diabetes and then adjust his medication, physical activity, and intake accordingly.

Samantha even joked about how he might have an easier time sticking to his health goals if he stared at the cashier's lovely eyes instead of at the croissant. Ted smiled as he recalled their conversation, how much they both laughed, and how good it felt to have Samantha understand him. He felt he could make a better decision and not just follow a thoughtless reflex. He excused himself from the order line, turned around, and walked down the block to a rival shop. He decided to start a new coffee-buying ritual: one without croissants, cake, or other baked goods. Ted felt proud. He made a mental note to e-mail Samantha and thank her for her help.

What If You Don't Like Your Patient?

Occasionally, we have to deal with patients we don't particularly like. For some reason that may be related to our own life experiences, they push our buttons. These feelings are perfectly normal, so don't dismiss them. Instead, use them diagnostically as a way to learn more about your patients and yourself. If Mrs. Leaf always had a lovely disposition, but suddenly comes to her appointment disgruntled and rude, SDR and then consider what physical and mental changes she may be experiencing. Is her glucose level abnormal? Is she becoming depressed? What else is happening in her life? If you feel uneasy around particular patients, your discomfort may highlight a behavior that they use with others. Note these red flags and investigate the physical, interpersonal, and emotional health issues they may represent.

Occasionally, our strong feelings can compromise the care we provide. We may not be able to connect with some patients, and they may have a harder time accepting help from us. John Bowlby's attachment theory offers a possible explanation for the negative encounters that occur between us and some of our more challenging patients. According to Bowlby, when all of us were young, our caretakers met our needs in ways that either comforted and reassured us or left us feeling anxious, lost, and unsupported. These early experiences helped us form "*enduring* cognitive models or 'maps' of caregiving that persist into adulthood" (Ciechanowski, 2002).

Adults with secure attachment histories are more at ease with those who reach out to assist them. Those with less or unresponsive early caregivers may have more difficulty trusting health care professionals, while individuals whose caregivers' attention was inconsistent try much harder to gain approval. These are the patients who may act more clingy and needy. Finally, individuals who experienced "overly critical or harsh rejecting caregiving" are more apt to demonstrate approach-avoidance behavior as a "manifestation of their fear of intimacy" (Ciechanowski, 2002). Their behaviors have both negative and positive aspects. For example, they may be excited to try what you suggest, but they won't actually do it. These different attachment responses are most apparent when the individuals need assistance, which is when most of us see our patients. When they meet with us, their attachment history helps them determine whether they can trust us as their caretakers and whether they feel they deserve to be helped. Understanding the basics of attachment theory can help us all see our patients' behaviors through a new lens and respond to them in a more positive way.

What About Our Own Attachment Issues?

We health care professionals have our own attachment histories, and develop attachments with our patients as well. We expect our patients to value us and turn to us when they are in need. We believe they should come to their appointments and follow the guidance we offer. At times, we may find ourselves trying too hard to get their approval. Our professional values also may be affected, if our attachment feelings start to unravel when patients miss multiple appointments. We may feel less committed or even threatened when patients bring conflicting opinions from other sources, such as the Internet. Instead of praising their efforts to find answers, which reflect the dedication they have to their health (and then discuss why the info may be incorrect), many of us express such strong negative responses that our patients become reluctant to share in the future:

> After Maxine shared an Internet article she printed out about hearing loss, which she was developing, her doctor went on a lengthy tirade about the unreliability of Internet medical information. Maxine felt hurt and dismissed. Today, she still looks things up on Webmd.com, a reliable website, but never shares it with her doctor. She also refrains from letting him know when she tries any of the suggested treatments posted on the site. Sadly, their relationship continues to suffer. Her doctor missed an opportunity to listen to Maxine's concern, acknowledge her efforts to learn more, and reflect back on the issues that worried her. His efforts could have positively affected the way she cared for her health.

Why Do They Push Our Buttons?

To understand and, hopefully, adjust the highly negative responses we have to some of our more frustrating patients, for their well-being and ours, we need to consider three things:

- Others may find these individuals frustrating too, so we shouldn't take their behavior personally.
- Their behavior may remind us of the behavior of others in our past or present.
- We may have a strong response because we possess the potential to behave the very same way.

"What we see in others may exist in ourselves, both the good and the bad. If you admire someone's courage, you notice it because it is in you as well" (Ford, 2010). What we dislike in others, we may dislike in ourselves. Think about a patient you find hard to tolerate. Identify what bothers you the most. For the sake of this discussion, let's say that you cringe every time you encounter Mrs. Groan's rudeness; it sets you on edge. You don't like how she speaks to you and ungratefully disputes everything you say. True, no one would appreciate that behavior, but why does it bother you so much? Why you feel this way may surprise you: You might dislike Mrs. Groan because her behavior reflects the rudeness you dislike in yourself. You may bend over backward to keep that side of yourself hidden, but it is possible that you have it. In fact, all the qualities we notice in others, both good and bad, may be qualities we have in varying amounts in ourselves.

To better accept or understand Mrs. Groan's behavior, try to reflect on and embrace that part of yourself. Look at the positive side of this hidden area of your personality—what Carl Jung refers to as our "shadow":

> Everyone carries a shadow, and the less it is embodied in the individual's conscious life, the blacker and denser it is. "If we are aware of a particular issue or pattern, one always has a chance to correct it . . . But if it is repressed and isolated from consciousness, it never gets corrected (Jung, 1975).

Let's give it a try:

- You dislike Mrs. Groan's rude behavior toward you and others in your office. She thinks she is entitled and throws her weight around each time she comes to see you—at least that is how you interpret her actions based on your past experiences.
- How are you like Mrs. Groan in this respect? Do you ever push your weight around? Do you have the tendency to be rude, but work hard to keep your behavior in line? We notice what is familiar. We recognize rudeness because it exists in us, we observed it in a family member, or we were the recipient of that behavior at some time in our past.

Let's return to Mrs. Groan. Unquestionably, her rudeness is at an unproductive level that you, and perhaps many others, feel needs to be toned down. But see how you feel about her and her behavior once you adopt a more compassionate attitude toward the rudeness you may have in yourself or in those who have behaved rudely toward you in the past. You may find that you suddenly see Mrs. Groan in a more accepting light—that she is in pain and her outbursts are her way of trying to control a life over which she feels she has little control. As you begin to understand her, you may feel yourself softening a little more each time you see her. Her strengths may become more apparent to you. Best of all, when your attitude shifts, Mrs. Groan's response to you may shift as well. Remember, communication is circular, so how you respond to one another is likely to change. As she becomes more receptive to your interest in her ideas, and enjoys improved health, you, hopefully, will get more enjoyment out of helping her meet her health goals.

This self-awareness can work with other people in your life as well. If you have a mother-in-law, for example, whose critical comments get on your nerves, recognize the highly critical behavior you have the potential to display. Does it ever surface or is it a behavior you battle to keep hidden? Regardless, it is possibly in you and that may be one reason why your mother-in-law's attacks hit you so hard. To move beyond this, consider how being critical of others works in your best interest, especially when it surfaces in a more gentle form. Your critical tendency, in measured doses, makes you a valuable team member because you always notice when something is missing. Embrace it; enjoy the fact that criticism, when used in the *right strength*, is beneficial. Here are steps you can take to do this activity:

1. Identify the quality you dislike in someone else.
2. Search for a similar quality you have or may have experienced when interacting with others.
3. Embrace its positive, balanced side.
4. Take a moment to feel some compassion for that person and whatever history or experience prompted this quality to surface.
5. Observe how your feelings about that person change. See if you can identify changes in your future interactions with others as well.

As you start to assume a more positive, growth-focused mind-set (Dweck, 2007) toward your patients, yourself, and others in your life (versus a fixed, perfection-focused mind-set), you may find that your approach to your work becomes more positive as well. For those patients who continue to bother you, breathe deeply and SDR.

When Should You Refer Your Patients to a Behavioral Health Professional?

According to the Diabetes Attitudes, Wishes, and Needs (DAWN) study, 85.2% of newly diagnosed patients with diabetes reported feeling shock, depression, anger, guilt, anxiety, and helplessness. For years after their diagnosis (up to 15 years, on average), patients reported that they still struggled with these feelings along with the "fear of complications and immediate social and psychological burdens of caring for diabetes" (Skovlund, 2005). Out of the

41% of individuals with diabetes who reported that they "had poor well-being, only 10% received any form of psychological treatment" (Peyrot, 2005).

There will be times when you see patients who are unable to move beyond their strong emotions. Is this the ideal time to refer them to a therapist? No. Did we surprise you with that response? We believe that patients who have access to qualified behavioral health professionals should meet with one *before* that moment occurs. Encourage your patients to have an introductory session with a therapist *as soon as possible after they are first diagnosed*. Everyone who has diabetes or another chronic medical issue should have the phone number of a trusted health psychology professional handy. Most people seek out a therapist when their problems become unmanageable. That isn't the time to shop around for a clinician who makes you feel comfortable.

Develop a relationship with one or more specialists in health psychology, such as a therapist, social worker, mental health counselor, family therapist, psychologist, or psychiatrist. Keep their business cards handy, so you can recommend them quickly and without reservation. Many therapists offer Skype sessions, which can be convenient for patients who, for a variety of reasons, can't meet with one in person. One source for online therapists who are familiar with diabetes-related issues is www.integrateddiabetes.com. All clinicians at this site have diabetes. It was created by the American Association of Diabetes Educators' 2014 Diabetes Educator of the Year, Gary Scheiner, MS, CDE. For patients with financial challenges, provide a list of low-cost or sliding-scale mental health resources in their area. The staff at any local hospital should be able to provide you with this information. You can contact a specialist in health psychology to help you handle difficult patient-related situations, group sessions, and even personal burnout.

How to Approach the Conversation

Some patients may not want to hear that you want them to meet with a mental health provider. Open the topic with a discussion of the following letter to help them understand why you are making this referral. Emphasize that you want all of your patients to live life as healthy individuals, not just as people who struggle with diabetes. Wendy often uses a light touch to soften a strong response. If after you suggest the referral, your patient asks, "Are you telling me I am crazy?" Wendy suggests you answer by saying, "Thanks for sharing your reaction so honestly. No, I think you'd be crazy *not* to go."

After their session, encourage your patients to share how everything went. A qualified therapist not only can help your patients develop more mutually supportive relationships with their loved ones, but also can help your patients relate better to their diagnosis, to its emotional challenges, to their new self-care responsibilities, and to you.

Dear Patient:

I would like you to meet with a therapist because—

- **I refer all of my patients to a therapist.** A therapist is a vital part of every diabetes team. If you have no emotional, social, family, or behavioral concerns right now, this referral can help you develop a relationship with someone who can assist you in the future.

- **How you think about your health can make a difference.** Your blood glucose can affect your mood and vice versa. A therapist can help you learn how to think about your health in a more positive way.

- **Living with diabetes can be stressful.** Your therapist can help you learn skills that enable you to interact with others better and handle stress, worries and fears more effectively.

- **A therapist can help you embrace yourself as a complete person**, not just as a person with diabetes.

    Name of therapist _____

    Phone _____

The Takeaway

To connect with your patients, listen, empathize, affirm, positively reframe (LEAP) and then refer.

4
For Your Toolbox, Part I

In this chapter, you will learn the following:

- Approaches you (and your patients) can use to enhance communication

Quite a few years ago, as a relatively inexperienced dietitian, Janis, one of our authors, attempted to counsel an obese, Black male with type 2 diabetes (T2D). After inquiring about the ethnic foods he enjoyed, a routine nutritional question, he suddenly banged on the desk and accused Janis of being a racist. She was stunned. Nothing like this had ever happened to her before. She apologized for any offensive comments she had made unknowingly, ended the session, and arranged for the gentleman to leave without paying the fee. Still shaken, Janis retold the incident to the referring endocrinologist who burst out laughing and admitted that he should have warned her as this was something that patient did quite often.

Years have passed and Janis now knows a lot more about how to handle challenging situations. Today, she wouldn't run from that gentleman's anger. She would want to know more about him and his anger and not end the session. She would invite him to consider that their interaction could still be worthwhile, despite his initial reaction or their dissimilar backgrounds. Janis would also share her insights with the endocrinologist, in a constructive and positive way, so both she and the doctor could work more effectively as a team.

- What can you do when tough emotions enter an appointment or counseling session?
- What can you do when your patient becomes extremely upset or angry, or you feel challenged?
- What can you do to help keep the session on track?

We introduced several options to you in earlier chapters, such as the stop, drop, and roll (SDR) intervention, which always should be the first action you take. The following are additional approaches you can use. Many are derived from interventions that are designed to be used by trained therapists, social workers, and other behavioral health professionals during single and multiple, hour-long therapy sessions. For the purposes of this book, however, we adapted these approaches into brief versions that don't require extensive training but do require some practice. With these abbreviated forms, you are less likely to achieve the cognitive change that happens with the skilled hand of a trained therapist, but they will help you show respect for your patients' feelings as well as your own and, hopefully, return the session back to its original focus. As you model these behaviors (and explain them briefly, if desired) your patients, hopefully, will feel motivated to try them with others in their lives also.

Anticipate (Plan Ahead)

Encourage your patients to mentally prepare for potentially emotional situations in their lives. If they attended their family's Thanksgiving dinner and were cornered by "Cousin Crystal" who questioned their food choices, help them anticipate what might happen when they see her again at the family's upcoming Christmas dinner. Many of the approaches we share in this book can help, such as deep breathing, self-talk, and visualization. Your patients also can prepare a few possible responses to say if the situation occurs again, such as, "Crystal, thanks for caring. I have a terrific dietitian who helps me make food decisions that are right for me."

If, in past sessions, certain patients cried when you discussed possible complications or triggered a strong emotional response in you when they shared falsified blood glucose test results, it makes sense to prepare yourself for the possibility of another emotional session. Anticipate the situation and calm yourself (SDR, breathe, self-talk, etc.) before you enter the exam room. When you and your patients anticipate potential emotional difficulties, you both should be better able to handle many tough situations when they arise.

A note about patient glucose self-reports: Patients who adjust their glucose data to meet certain criteria may do so for a variety of reasons. They may not want to share what's really going on in their lives, they may feel the need to be perfect in this area, they may not want family members to see how much they are struggling, or they may simply have forgotten to do them and rushed to jot something down on their way to the appointment to avoid disappointing you.

They also may be responding to messages you communicate. Do you only recognize results and forget to praise their efforts? Do you shake your head in disapproval, circle "bad" numbers with a bright colored pen, or raise your eyebrows in dismay when you see less-than-optimal results? Anticipate what you may communicate with your words and actions and try to adjust your message before you meet with these patients in the future.

Affirm (Normalize and Validate)

What your patients feel and do is not unusual; others act and feel the same way too. If you fly to New York City in the dead of winter, for example, you will feel cold when you take your first step outside of the airport. All of your fellow passengers will feel that way too. They may not act on the feeling in the same way, but you likely won't be the only one who acts on their feelings in that respect either. Some will button up their warm coats more tightly, whereas others will leave their coats open, brave the cold, and continue to feel miserable. Let your patients know that their feelings and behaviors are a normal part of being human. Remember this for yourself as well. Even though you are a professional, at times you will experience feelings or act in ways that don't seem very professional (i.e., jealousy, anger or yelling, forgetting, etc.) For more information on affirming, see Chapter 3.

Show Appreciation

People feel more positive when they know their efforts are appreciated. A word or two of appreciation can help your patients feel comfortable and more at ease with their actions:

Kim hands you her blood glucose record. She worries that you will be upset by what you see. She believes the results are not good and expects to be criticized for them. You respond with a big smile and say, "Kim, thank you for bringing this today. I know that some of your results fell outside of your target range, but you didn't seem to let them discourage you—you still continued to check your blood at the times we discussed. This information helps us both understand your needs better.

When a patient or co-worker criticizes you, respond with a message of appreciation instead of anger or frustration: "Thanks for letting me know. I didn't realize that bothered you so much." This response will surprise them if they expected a battle. You acknowledged that person's feelings and sent a respectful message in return. When you do this, you don't necessarily admit to any wrongdoing, but you do show that you now realize that your actions bothered them. Appreciation also can come in the form of compliments. Accept good feelings your patients' positive comments prompt in you. Acknowledge their comments by thanking them. Say, "Thank you. That feels so nice. You made my day." Don't be afraid to congratulate yourself when you did something well. You deserve the praise.

Assertive Language

Assertive language helps you focus on specific goals, while showing empathy for the listener. Those who use it converse in a rational, calm, honest, and direct way. They don't yell, blame, respond aggressively, or remain passive when it is important to speak up. Assertive comments focus on your personal feelings and needs. It uses assertive and empathic "I" language rather than blaming and accusatory "You" language.

Accusatory "You" Language

Accusatory "you" language includes statements like the following: "*You* have to stop ignoring my recommendations." Or "Please stop bringing me articles *you* find on the Internet. *You* aren't going to find any valuable medical advice there." Read these sentences and consider how you might react if someone said them to you. Would you respond with support or feel prompted to fight back?

Assertive, Empathic "I" Language

Assertive, empathic "I" language includes statements like the following: "*I believe* you care about your health. When you don't check your blood, *I feel* frustrated. I need that information so I can help you." Or "*I think* you want my guidance, but *I feel* like that isn't the case when you repeatedly cancel your appointments. *I am glad* you are here today. What would make it easier for you to keep your appointments?" (Repeat the message as needed without escalating your feelings.) How would you feel if someone made those comments to you? The attack language is gone. The speaker opens by saying how much he supports and appreciates your concern and then let's you know how it makes *him* feel. Do you feel more inclined to continue the conversation and solve the problem? Use assertive language in your own life. See how others respond when you do. When you feel comfortable with it, help your patients use it in tough situations that arise. Role-play challenging interactions with them so that they can experiment with different ways to word their messages. Let them know they have a voice and will get far better results when they use it effectively, empathically, and assertively.

Set Boundaries

If necessary, let your patients know they can establish clear boundaries for themselves and their diabetes. They do not have to tell everyone they know about their disease; whom they tell is a personal decision. They should, however, disclose their medical needs to those who can help them if an emergency arises, such as a roommate or co-worker. It is also helpful to disclose this information to their employer. They aren't legally obligated to do so, but if they choose not to tell, they may lose certain workplace discrimination protections (Davidson, 2012). It's not helpful to keep diabetes under wraps because of feelings of shame. Some patients might want to do so because they desire privacy. Role-play mock interactions so they can practice responding to those who ask about their disease. Suggest they say, "Thanks for taking the time to think about me. I have a great medical team and am on top of my diabetes." If some of your patients don't feel comfortable setting boundaries, encourage them to meet with the therapist on your team to learn how to do so.

As a health care professional, you also benefit from having clear boundaries. Clearly distinguish when you are on and off duty and when you are doing too much or too little for your patients. When work and private life boundaries become blurred, you are at greater risk for developing professional burnout.

Cognitive Restructuring

"For there is nothing either good or bad, but thinking makes it so.
—*Hamlet*, Act 2, Scene 2, 239–251

We can *choose* how we perceive the events in our lives. A delay in our schedule doesn't have to be the end of the world. An abnormal blood glucose level doesn't have to be a sign of failure. We don't have to accept our negative thoughts as truths. Following are two steps you can take to help alter the way you think about different situations (Boyes, 2013).

Step 1. Thought-Tracking

Keep track of any cognitive distortions you make for an entire week. A cognitive distortion is any thought that doesn't accurately represent reality. For example, you always may expect the worst to happen when it rarely does. When negative thoughts come to mind, think for a moment about how and where you learned this response. Then consider how else you could perceive the situation. Ask yourself, "What's the worst that could happen?" "What's the best that could happen?" and "What is most likely to happen?" You have the power to change how you feel and respond.

Step 2. Monitor the Accuracy of Your Thoughts

How often did any of your negative thoughts come true? Keep track and check your results. If you think negatively about things that usually turn out well, you, hopefully, will see that your predictions are not always accurate. If negative thinking continues to bother your patients (or you), have them meet with the behavioral health specialist on your team for additional guidance.

Collaborative Conversation

Collaborative conversations happen between individuals who genuinely want to know and understand one another. They come together without prejudgments or assumptions. Kellie Rodriguez, MSN, CDE, CPT, former director of educational services at Miami's Diabetes Research Institute, converses this way with all of her patients. She views each meeting as a platonic "date" during which she tries to get to know her patients as individuals. She shares a little of herself as well. To be an effective educator, Kellie tries to "understand how diabetes navigates through [my patient's] life and how their life navigates its way through diabetes." She often asks, "Who are you? What does your life involve? What makes you smile?" She uses her patients' responses to help them find motivation that can support their desire to participate in more positive health behaviors. She finds that this collaborative approach helps build rapport and trust, which are "essential ingredients to a healthy, mutually respectful health care provider/patient relationship." Engage in collaborative conversations with patients, colleagues, family, and friends. When you show sincere interest in what another person has to say, you connect on a far deeper level (Kellie Rodriguez, e-mail message to author, October 8, 2013).

Behavioral Health Screening

Keep a reliable depression-screening tool in your office and have your patients complete it. Follow up with your patients by referring them to the behavioral health professional on your team. Discuss the referral letter at the end of Chapter 3 to help them understand why you are asking them to go. Use the short version of the Problem Areas in Diabetes Scale for diabetes-related distress (McGuire, 2010), our progress scale, and inquire about such issues as anxiety, substance abuse, eating disorders, sexual functioning, sleep disorders, attention deficit–hyperactivity disorder, and tobacco cessation when the need arises.

Education

Most people feel uncomfortable about the unknown. When you provide additional facts about a particular issue or concern, your patients are more likely to feel at ease. It also arms them with information they can share with relatives and friends who urge them to behave in ways that may not be beneficial to their health. But don't ask them to simply pick up an educational brochure as they leave the office. Try to make all of these educational moments interactive. Engage your patients in a discussion about their concerns. If they are willing, invite them to summarize what they know about the topic in a sentence or two. You might be surprised by how much they know. This exchange will give you an opportunity to gently correct any misinformation they share. If appropriate, use a bit of humor to lighten the discussion. Humor helps reduce discomfort (Bennett, 2008) and facilitates emotional connection and learning. You can educate your colleagues, friends, and family about the approaches you learn in this book.

Empathic Confrontation

At some point, you may have to confront a few of your patients about their ineffective health decisions. When you do, be empathic: Ask what prompted them to make these decisions then listen to their responses. Their reasons may surprise you. Wendy met with a young man who kept "forgetting" to check his blood glucose level. His parents were sure that he was being an irresponsible teen. But they were mistaken. When Wendy spoke to the young man privately, he shared that he was skipping his blood tests to protect his mother. She always got upset when his meter showed a high number, so he decided to spare her and not to check his blood anymore. His decision, although misguided, was a thoughtful example of "intelligent nonadherence" (Hindi-Alexander, 1987); he made a conscious choice not to follow an important health directive. When you interact with your patients with empathy, you invite honest interaction. Come to each confrontation with an open heart and mind.

Empathic Listening: LEAP

Listen to your patients without judging them. Be curious. Don't anticipate what their responses might be. Your patients have waited a long time to see you and now deserve to be the focus of your *undivided* attention, even if your time together is limited. Harville Hendrix, cocreator of Imago Relationship Therapy, defines empathy as "the ability to understand what another person is experiencing even though you have not had that identical experience" (Hendrix, 2008). When you listen empathically, your patients will feel that you "get" them. The four steps to empathic listening (as described in Chapter 3) are LEAP:

1. Listen with sincere curiosity.
2. Empathize—explore and try to understand what matters to them.
3. Affirm that their feeling and behavior is common (or has been done by others at some point in time).
4. Positively reframe—share a more upbeat perspective.

Encouragement

As a health care professional, you probably had at least one person encourage you to become the individual you are today. It might have been a teacher, relative, trusted colleague, or friend. Think of how their words and unshakable support made you feel, especially when times got tough. It isn't easy to live with diabetes. Be one of the special people in your patients' lives and offer them kind and generous words of encouragement that reflect the strengths you see. Your words not only can help them get through trying times but also can introduce them to a positive perspective they can reflect on when you are not around.

Externalizing Conversations

This interaction comes from narrative therapy, an innovative counseling approach developed by Michael White and David Epston (White, 2007). Externalizing conversations encourage people to separate themselves from the problems in their lives. Once they achieve this, they can see their challenging issues from a new perspective and identify ways to deal with them. To do this, follow three steps:

1. Identify the problem and personify it (give it a name and a color, or refer to it as a person).
2. Search for exceptions (times when the problem doesn't exist).
3. Use the exceptions to identify solutions.

Here is how Janis used this approach with one of her patients:

Step 1. Identify the Problem and Personify It

"Lynn" is a 65-year-old White female with T2D. She kept gaining weight, which has made her diabetes difficult to manage. She felt like a failure because she was unable to control her appetite. Her husband was furious with her behavior, and her doctor said that he was ready to give up on her. Janis, her diabetes educator, met with Lynn and said that she was not the problem, her hunger was. She asked her to assign her hunger a name and a color. Lynn called it "Red Fred."

Step 2. Search for Exceptions

Janis asked Lynn to identify times when "Red Fred" didn't bother her—when "he" didn't prompt her to overeat. When could Lynn push "him" away? Lynn responded, "Red Fred doesn't bother me when I work on the computer or when I walk outside. I don't feel hungry at those times." Janis commented on Lynn's response: "At first, you said that you have no control over your hunger, but that isn't true. You don't eat when you work on the computer or when you walk outside. At those times, you control Red Fred quite well. You are more powerful than 'he' is when you do those things."

Step 3. Identify Solutions

Janis asked Lynn to identify more times when she successfully pushed Red Fred away and encouraged her to gradually add them to her day. Lynn decided to walk every morning for 15 minutes. Slowly, she added additional positive behaviors to her schedule. After several weeks, she stopped overeating and began to lose weight. Lynn, her husband, her doctor, and Janis were thrilled.

Feelings Pass

Many patients and professionals feel overwhelmed by certain feelings. We can feel paralyzed and believe that our feelings will last forever. Help your patients visualize the passing of their emotions. Follow these steps to help them do this:

1. Identify the feeling
2. Affirm the feeling
3. Visualize the feeling passing

Consider the following example: Sue learns that she must start using insulin and begins to sob.

1. **You say:** "I see that this really upsets you." "What bothers you the most?" (*Identify.*) Sue says she is afraid of the pain.
2. **You respond:** "Many of my patients feel afraid at first, just like you do. (*Affirm that it's typical.*) But they all say that the shots don't really hurt. They are also so impressed with how well their insulin works that they want to know why I didn't have them start it sooner.
3. **You continue:** "Picture yourself successfully using insulin. Now, picture yourself coming back to see me (or e-mail me) to say you wish I had started you on insulin sooner, too. (*Visualize.*)

Forgiveness

The act of forgiving can be transformative and healing. Forgiveness "is a decision to let go of resentment and thoughts of revenge" (Mayo Clinic, 2011). It doesn't mean endorsing or ignoring hurtful actions. Those responsible must still accept responsibility for their behavior. When patients forgive the medical specialist who initially misdiagnosed them, relatives who insulted them, and even themselves for not taking care of their diabetes as well as they believe they should have, they can move forward. When people let go of their "grudges and bitterness," they have a greater opportunity to enjoy more meaningful relationships. Medically, their blood pressure may improve, they may feel less depressed, and they may start to enjoy a less stressful life (Mayo Clinic, 2011).

As a health care provider, you may feel angry about patients who are disrespectful, about colleagues who take credit for your ideas, and even about your own medical misjudgments. Adopt a forgiving attitude towards others as well as yourself and enjoy the mental and physical benefits.

Gratitude

When any of your patients lose certain abilities as a result of diabetes-related complications, you may be tempted to ask them to appreciate all they are still able to do. Give into that temptation only after you first acknowledge their loss. If you neglect to do so, your comments can come across as dismissive. When you encourage your patients to see the glass as "half-full" you help them more than you think. People who feel grateful adapt more easily to challenges, experience reduced stress, and enjoy improved sleep (Wood, 2010). Their feelings of gratitude also can make your job easier as those who feel gratitude are more likely to notice how hard you try to help them (McCullough, 2001).

In your workplace, take a few extra moments to thank co-workers and colleagues for what they do. Your actions are a worthwhile investment in the future as people who aren't thanked for their efforts are "less likely to provide help in the future" (Wood, 2010).

Humor

Dr. Patch Adams, the "clown" doctor played by Robin Williams in the film, *Patch Adams*, urges us all to infuse our practices with humor. According to Adams (2002) adding humor is easy to do if you approach your patients with compassion. "If a patient perceives you love them, they will forgive (even delight in) any humorous experiences you share." According to Penson (2005) humor helps health care professionals "foster deeper, more trusting relationships with their patients" and can "help narrow interpersonal and cultural gaps by aiding doctor-patient communication." Humor also helps relieve any tension that may exist when you discuss sensitive subjects. But it can be misused, so monitor your patients' reactions closely. If they feel defensive, they may be insulted by your attempts to point out the lighter side of their concerns. Certainly don't make any jokes at anyone's expense. Introduce humor into a session slowly. Wendy completed her doctoral dissertation on "Humor as a Coping Mechanism with Diabetes." When people ask, "Is your diabetes contagious?" She suggests they say, "Thanks for asking. If I don't like you, it is!"

Know Your History (Transference)

How we perceive verbal and nonverbal messages often has a lot to do with our past experiences. You may be familiar with the term "transference." Transference happens when we unconsciously apply a feeling from our past to someone in our current lives. For instance, if your mother used food to show love, the associate who brings cookies to the office may look better in your eyes. You are "transferring" your loving, food-related memory to your present situation. On the other hand, someone whose mother forced them to eat everything on their plate each evening may have a more negative response to the co-worker who arrives carrying cookies. If Cindy hated being yelled at by her parents to clean her room, she might start to seethe when her office mate innocently asks her to tidy up a shared cabinet or shelf. Pay attention to how your personal history colors the way you interpret the actions of others. If you react strongly to a certain message or event and don't know why, slow down and consider your history. Be aware if you tend to be reactive to or become inhibited by people's ages, genders, sexual orientation, race, or religion and then SDR.

Letter Writing and Journaling

If you or your patients are upset about a certain topic, pull out a sheet of paper, gather your angry thoughts and write a letter to the issue.

- Dear Diabetes . . .
- Dear boss who keeps threatening to fire me . . .
- Dear co-worker who moves my chair whenever I'm away from my desk . . . etc.

Accurate spelling and grammar are optional—you can write anything you like, using any words you choose. When done, put the paper away or tear it up, and observe how you feel. You don't have to show anyone what you write. Writing clarifies your feelings and can change the way you perceive a particular issue. It also enables you to get your strong feelings out in the open and then, at a later point, reread it and see how much you have changed. Expressive writing in a journal can improve your mood, emotional and physical symptoms, and strengthen your immune system (Baikie, 2005).

Miracle Question—Abbreviated

This solution-focused family therapy approach helps patients who feel negatively about certain areas of their lives, or about their lives as a whole, by helping them clarify what they want so that they can identify a new set of goals. To use this approach, ask the following question: "If you went to sleep tonight and a miracle happened—the problem(s) you are struggling with disappeared— what one or two ways would tomorrow be different? A therapist who uses this technique would walk your patient, slowly and methodically, through each moment of the day. You don't have that much time, but you can ask this question to learn what type of change your patients want in their lives. Once you get their response, help them find a way to include that change in their lives.

Joan, you may recall, dropped out of her aerobics class because of her neuropathy pain. If you ask her the miracle question, she might say, "If I woke up and my leg pain was gone, I would run over to my aerobics class and dance again with my friends." Joan obviously wants to be active again and see her friends. Ask if she could try any other aerobics classes. Perhaps the aerobics' center offers chair-dancing (seated aerobics) classes. Or, if her health allows, maybe she could join a water aerobics class. If she misses her workout buddies, invite her to consider other ways to be with them. Maybe they could join her for lunch once a month. A few minutes of brainstorming can open your patients up to possibilities they never considered before. These alternate options can help them feel less trapped by their problems.

You can use the miracle question with your own negative feelings as well. Consider how your day would change if the issues that bother you today suddenly were resolved. How would tomorrow be different from today? Try to transform some of the changes into reality.

Motivational Interviewing

Motivational interviewing is a collaborative approach that takes a great deal of training to learn to do correctly. Many experts have recommended it for all patients, especially those who are ambivalent about making changes. MI helps patients move through the following stages of readiness:

- **Precontemplation:** Not yet ready to consider any change
- **Contemplation:** Thinking about making a change within the next 6 months
- **Preparation:** Getting ready to make a change within the next 30 days
- **Action:** Currently attempting the new behavior
- **Maintenance:** 60 or more days after making the change

Once you identify a patient's stage, empower him or her to take "small action steps" that best suit his or her current level (Hodorowicz, 2013). Many excellent books have been written about MI. Explore this topic if you are interested in using it in your practice.

The Takeaway

Try these approaches with your patients and others in your life. Read Chapter 5 for additional suggestions.

5
For Your Toolbox, Part II

I n this chapter, you will continue to learn the following:

- More approaches you (and your patients) can use to enhance communication

Naming: Point It Out

After you SDR, which should always be the first step you take, identify any emotions you sense in the room. When you do this, it enables you to connect empathically with your patients (friend, partner, co-worker, etc.) and validate their feelings. People respond positively when their feelings are acknowledged without judgment (remember Carl Rogers from Chapter 3). If Susan appears nervous, name what you think you see and invite her to confirm or deny your observation: "Susan, you seem uneasy today. How are you feeling?" If John appears distracted during your presentation on carbohydrate counting, don't ignore his behavior. Point it out: "John, I see that you keep looking around the room. What's on your mind? Would you like me to stop for a moment? Naming may sound like a simple task, but it can be hard to do at first. As a sensitive health provider, you already respond to emotions that arise: When your patients become frustrated, you slow down your explanation or repeat what you just said to ensure that they understand your message. Now add the next step and point out what you see so they can share their thoughts. Describe the emotion and then observe how your patients respond. For example: "You seem very quiet today, Tim. I seem to be the only one doing any of the talking." Then wait silently (yes, it's hard to do!) and let Tim share his thoughts about your comment.

Network

Each of us has a network of colleagues and experts. Maintain an active referral list of experts on your team to whom you and your patients can turn for support and guidance. Assist those who reach out to you. Diabetes care takes a village for patients *and* professionals.

Positively Reframe

When patients or others around you focus on a negative thought, take the time to acknowledge and understand their concerns. After you have done that, let them know that there may be other ways to look at their situation. They can *choose* to see troubling issues in a different, more upbeat way. A positive reframe is a way to perceive a feeling or situation from a more upbeat perspective. Developing diabetes, for example, which is a devastating diagnosis, is seen by some as a "gift" that motivates them to live a healthier life. Exercise can be seen as a way to make new friends, reduce stress, and feel better. Plateauing during a weight loss attempt is evidence that the dieter is maintaining, not gaining, which is definitely worthy of praise. When people view things in a more positive way, they can become more hopeful. To help your patients think about the challenges in their lives from a more positive perspective, ask them to make a list of adjectives and come up with a positive reframe for each of them, such as the following:

- Quiet vs. thoughtful
- Stubborn vs. determined
- Loud and exuberant vs. joyful
- Afraid vs. cautious
- Stressful vs. stimulating
- Annoying vs. loves being with you

When dealing with patients with varying backgrounds, don't forget that their culture can play a role in how they view their situation (Kim, 2012).

See your patients, co-workers, friends, and loved ones as individuals and appreciate that they may not always have the same perspective you do. For more on this topic, see Chapter 3.

Prayer and Spirituality

"When fear knocks, let faith answer," says Robin Roberts, co-host of ABC's Good Morning America who underwent a life-saving bone marrow transplant. For religious and spiritually connected patients, such as Roberts, faith provides a great deal of support. "Spirituality can exert a tremendous impact on one's health and promote recovery from trauma and illness" (Torosian, 2005). For some people, the repetitious nature of prayer along with its positive messages are both meditative and uplifting (Kaplan, 1995). Those who aren't particularly religious or spiritual might consider the alternative perspective of Marya Hornbacher, author of *Waiting: A Nonbeliever's Higher Power*: "When I speak of spirit, I am not speaking of something related to or given by a force outside ourselves . . . I am speaking of the human *spirit* that exists in each of us" (Hornbacher, 2011).

Prayer not only can help some individuals handle personal struggles, but it also can help them with communal slights as well. According to a University of Michigan study, subjects who prayed for those who angered them enjoyed reduced feelings of anger and aggression (Bremner, 2011). If you aren't particularly spiritual or religious, don't underestimate the power of your patients' belief systems to help them cope with their diagnosis and with the challenges of self-care. Encourage them to explore what helped them in the past and what supports them today. If you are religious or spiritual, take care not to impose your perspective.

Reinforcing

The notion that it takes 21–28 days to learn a new habit has been batted around in the literature for quite some time (Goetzke, 2010). But the reality is that it probably takes much longer. Researchers in the United Kingdom found that it took between 18 and 254 days to establish a new habit (Lally, 2010). So don't give up when your patients don't pick up a healthful habit quickly. New behaviors take time to acquire and may need additional reinforcement. Hopefully, you also will go easier on yourself. Forgive yourself for failing to habituate a new, healthy behavior within 28 days. You aren't a failure, you just haven't reached your personal number of habit-forming days. (*Positive reframe!*) Continue to reinforce the positive behaviors you want to adopt and give yourself plenty of time to achieve that goal.

Reprioritizing

Many people feel stressed when their "to-do list" grows too large. Your patients easily can become overwhelmed with all they must do to care for their diabetes, and you may feel buried under your own work and health obligations. When this happens, reprioritize your list so the most critical tasks aren't missed. Janis uses the following circles activity to help her patients organize their priorities:

1. Draw a small, medium, and large circle on a sheet of paper.
2. Ask your patients to list the tasks they need to do each day (or week, etc.).
3. As they list each task, have them write it down in the circle that represents its importance. Small = minimal importance; medium = more important; large = very important.
4. Brainstorm ways to incorporate the more pressing tasks into their lives.

Role-Play

Because of their particular health needs, people with diabetes sometimes must engage in uncomfortable conversations. Like the employee who wants to ask his co-workers to keep their holiday treats farther away from his desk. Or the young woman who doesn't know how to tell her date she has diabetes. Help your patients gain conversational confidence by role-playing these and other similar situations. As you act out the event, encourage your patients to try different ways to word their messages. Offer a variety of emotional responses (surprised, supportive, insulted, etc.) so your patients can prepare themselves to react respectfully if the conversation doesn't go as anticipated. Role-playing helps patients feel more confident about engaging in these interactions. "Role-playing is a great way to gain insight into yourself and others. It can help you become more sensitive to the positions of others and help you understand how others see you as well as improve your confidence" (Zwolinski, 2011).

Scaling Questions

Scaling questions, a solution-focused therapy approach, invites individuals to "quantify their own perception of a situation" using a scale from 1 to 10 (Goldenberg, 2008). This activity can be especially eye-opening to patients who feel disappointed about their perceived lack of progress. This approach is frequently used in MI. In the following example, Tom discusses his daily walking with his educator:

Tom: I want to quit. I don't think I want to walk anymore.

Educator: Tom, before you decide to quit, let's first see if you gained anything from walking. On a scale of 1 to 10, how would you rank the changes you've experienced since you started? Let's have 1 represent absolutely no change and 10 represent really great improvements.

Tom: Well, my clothes are fitting more loosely and my morning blood glucose results have improved. I guess I would rate the changes at a 6.

Educator: A 6? That's quite high. How come you didn't rank it a 4 or 5?

Tom: A 4 wouldn't be high enough. I am really seeing improvements. I guess I should stay the course, huh?

Educator: Tom, it is up to you to continue. I'm not going to drag you out of bed each morning so you can walk! But, your improvements are impressive. Do you see that? What do you think it would take for you to rank your changes a 7 or 8?

Tom: Right now, I'm walking 15 minutes every morning. I could increase my walking to 30 minutes. I think I'd like to try that.

Search for Exceptions

This approach is especially helpful when patients use all-or-nothing types of phrases, such as "I never" or "I always." For example, Tammy says that she *always* overeats. Ask whether that is true. Does she really overeat at *every* meal, *every* day? Let her consider her schedule and respond with additional clarity. She may tell you that she doesn't overeat at breakfast or lunch, but she usually does overeat at dinner. Now she has identified some exceptions to her "always overeats" statement. Praise those moments as evidence that she has some control over her eating. This recognition of her actual behavior may help her gain the confidence she needs to tackle other challenges. For additional information about this approach, see Externalizing Conversations in Chapter 4.

Self-Compassion

Diabetes and perfection don't go together. Mistakes are opportunities for growth. Most of us learn more from things that don't go well than from those that go smoothly. As health care providers, we know that our patients can follow every directive perfectly, yet they still may have a fluctuating blood glucose level or other diabetes-related problem. Encourage your patients to treat themselves with compassion. "Self-compassionate people recognize that being imperfect, failing, and experiencing life difficulties is inevitable" (Neff, 2011). Give them permission to be human. Kristin Neff, author of *Self-Compassion: Stop Beating Yourself Up and Leave Insecurity Behind*, encourages people to go easy on themselves when things don't go right: "Self-compassion entails being warm and understanding toward ourselves when we suffer, fail, or feel inadequate, rather than ignoring our pain or flagellating ourselves with self-criticism." If we believe that we should always get what we want and deserve, we are setting ourselves up for a lifetime of frustration. Instead, help your patients— and yourself—view each mistake as a learning opportunity (*positive reframe*). When we learn, we grow.

Self-Disclosure

Several years ago, Janis went to her physician for a regular checkup. While there, she mentioned that she had started working as a therapist as well as a diabetes educator. Her doctor took her comment as an invitation to share his personal battle with depression. He then spent the brief time they had together chatting about the medications he had tried and the experts he had seen. At the end of the appointment, Janis was tempted to send him a bill for her counseling services.

When Is It Okay to Share a Personal Story With A Patient?

Some believe that personal disclosure is never appropriate (De Jong, 2008), whereas others think that it can be beneficial. For example, when faced with a dilemma, a patient may look to you for guidance and ask, "What would you do?" Your personal response could significantly reduce his or her anxiety (Nisselle, 2004). If you are tempted to self-disclose, evaluate your motivations before doing so. If you want to share a particular success story to impress your patients, reconsider. Your sharing will be all about you and not about them. If your tale is a precautionary one, "Don't go hiking without snacks, I once did that and boy, was I sorry!" then your story could be helpful. If you choose to disclose, keep your comments brief and always consider how your patient might think and feel after hearing what you say. You certainly don't want to say too much about poor decisions you make or struggles you have with your staff. If you do, your patients may lose confidence in your abilities.

Self-Talk

In Chapter 1, we introduced you to Peggy who had a hard time managing her negative internal messages. We said it was possible to transform negative messages into more positive ones and that we each had the power to do that. Now, let's talk about how that can be done. One way to achieve this is to shine a spotlight on these dark thoughts and see them for what they usually are: inaccurate interpretations of reality. A colleague of ours recently submitted a manuscript for publication. Multiple experts reviewed it and praised it highly. But one publishing assistant demanded that a particular chapter be rewritten multiple times. "It's still not there yet," the staff member said. Our colleague was distraught. She said, "I'm obviously a terrible writer! I should just give up." We challenged this and asked, "Are you really a bad writer?" The experts loved her writing. Other publishers raved about her work. It was this individual, alone, who took issue with a single chapter. Once we pointed that out to her, the light went on—she wasn't in an all-or-nothing" situation. She was a wonderful writer who could possibly learn something new from the assistant. She felt relieved and decided to talk to the publishing assistant that afternoon and hear what she had to say.

Invite your patients (and yourself) to challenge the accuracy of negative messages they receive from others as well as from themselves. Many times, negative messages say more about the sender than the receiver. Another option is to use the thought-tracking technique we suggested in the Cognitive Restructuring in Chapter 4. That method can help as well. Again, if negative self- talk continues to interfere with your life or the lives of your patients, meet with the behavioral health expert on your team for additional guidance.

Silence

Have you ever asked a question and your patient just sat there without saying a word? When a patient is silent, it is tempting to rush in and fill the conversational void. But don't do that. Your patient might be "sorting out his or her thoughts, is confused or angry about the situation just described, or is simply taking a short breather from the work at hand" (De Jong, 2008). When people have a lot on their minds, they often need a moment or two to consider what they'd like to share. If you jump in too soon, you take away the moment your patient may need to get up the courage to tell you something important. When in doubt, ask: "Is there something you would like to say?" or "You look like you are thinking about something important." If they answer no, stay quiet for a moment to see whether they respond. If not, move on and remind them that you always are willing to listen to any concerns or doubts they may have.

Slow Down (Mindfulness)

Where's the fire, what's the hurry about?
You'd better cool it off before you burn it out
You got so much to do and
Only so many hours in a day
—Billy Joel, "Vienna," *The Stranger* (1977)

In Chapter 1, we introduced mindfulness as a way to be mentally present throughout your day. But mindfulness offers an additional benefit: It can slow down time, or at least your perception of it. As a child, why did summer days drag on and on, yet now you barely have enough time to accomplish all you want to do each day? Time isn't changing, the way you perceive it is. David Eagleman, a neuroscientist, refers to time perception as a "rubbery thing" that speeds up or slows down depending on our level of "mental engagement" (Gregoire, 2013). To slow down time, pay closer attention to everything that happens around you. According to Eagleman, "The more detailed the memory, the longer the moment seems to last." When you meet with your patients, slow down. If your thoughts race when you are with your patients, you are less likely to notice their feelings, especially if they surface in subtle ways: The way their eyes moisten when they mention a loved one who upsets them or the way they clear their throats when they tell you how hard it is to inject their medication each morning. Be there for your patients and their emotional needs as well as their physical ones. And see how much more pleasure you get out of life when you pay more attention to all that is around you.

Strength-Based Questions

"Motivation increases when there is a consistent focus on strengths" (De Jong, 2008). People tend to dwell on their shortcomings, so help your patients focus on their strengths instead. Strength-based questions focus on strengths, not deficits. They enhance our enthusiasm and motivation. When we focus on our strengths, we change how we perceive ourselves, our patients, members of our families, and colleagues. All individuals have strengths they can tap into to help solve their problems. When you meet patients who believe they can't do something, steer the conversation away from their deficits and focus on their strengths. Be generous and do that for yourself as well. The following are two different conversations Linda had with her diabetes educator, Dave. One is deficit-focused and the other is strengths-focused.

Deficit-Focused Conversation

Consider the following deficit-focused conversation:

Dave: Linda, are you physically active?

Linda: I walked regularly for a few months, but I stopped quite a while ago.

Dave: What happened? Why did you stop? (*Focusing on her deficits.*)

Linda: Oh, I give up on everything. I'm hopeless. (*Linda reminds herself of her weaknesses.*)

Dave: Could you try starting again?

Linda: No, I really don't think so.

Strengths-Focused Conversation

Compare the previous conversation with this strengths-focused conversation:

Dave: Linda, are you physically active?

Linda: I walked regularly for a few months, but I stopped quite a while ago.

Dave: Great! You walked for a few months. That's impressive. How were you able to do that?" (*Focusing on her strengths.*)

Linda: I made time for it on my days off. I set my alarm and got out of the house early. I enjoyed it. I felt so healthy and had great blood glucose readings. Everyone commented on how much energy I had. I really should start again.

Dave: You did it once. How could you start doing it again?

Linda: I could start by setting my alarm again. I could also see if my sister wants to join me on one of the mornings. She lives down the block. If she can't come, I could phone her while I walk. We chat every morning. I could walk while I do that.

Dave: Great. You came up with a really good plan. E-mail the office to let me know how things go. I like hearing from my patients!

At the end of the deficit-focused exchange, Linda gave up. She remembered how much she lacked and felt it impossible to adopt this healthy behavior. The strength-focused conversation ended with Linda's commitment to try again in a very specific way.

Stop, Drop, and Roll

The stop, drop, and roll (SDR) intervention always should be the *first* action you take when you have or encounter a strong emotion. We discussed this option in Chapter 1, so take the following as a reminder. Just as you need to put on your oxygen mask before assisting others on an airplane, you must take care of your emotional needs before you help your patients deal with theirs:

1. Stop (If you find it helpful, visualize a red stop sign). Stop what you are doing and breathe. Then identify (name) the negative thought you just received from your critical inner voice.
2. Drop. Drop the negative message about yourself or your patient and adopt a calmer, more generous, and compassionate one.
3. Roll. Roll forward with your new compassionate message to yourself and your patient. Repeat steps 1 and 2 as needed if your first attempt is unsuccessful.

Stories

When patients arrive upset or become emotional during a session, invite them to share what happened. When people tell their stories out loud, they can consider them from a fresh perspective. "Stories help us smooth out some of the decisions we have made and create something that is meaningful and sensible out of the chaos of our lives" (Dingfelder, 2011). Telling stories is not only beneficial for your patients. You can learn a great deal from what they say. When people tell stories, they mention details that have meaning for them.

If they talk about the day they forgot to bring their insulin to an event, for example, ask what they learned from that experience and point out how that situation can remind them to be prepared. If they tell you about a time they believe they were treated badly by a relative, listen empathically, and consider that some of their relationships may be less supportive, they may feel defensive, or they may need to become more adept at using assertive language (see Chapter 4).

Because your time is limited, encourage patients to limit each story to a set length and to express what they believe they learned from the experience. Look at your patients' stories as part of their treatment and not a waste of valuable time. It is heartwarming to hear patients share what is going well in their lives. But don't miss out on the wealth of information you can learn from situations that don't go as planned. Alternatively, if you ignore how they feel, they may be so distracted by their thoughts that they pay less attention to what you have to offer. If their story has a humorous twist, laugh with them and remind them how much they probably will enjoy talking about a future awkward or uncomfortable situation. If appropriate, share stories of your own to help guide your patients or illustrate a particular point (see the section Self-Disclosure).

Summarizing (Reflecting)

When you occasionally reflect and summarize what your patients tell you, you communicate your desire to understand their lives and their needs. Reflecting happens when you repeat someone's message back to them (in your own words) to confirm that you heard their story accurately. It's very validating. You also can ask them to summarize the messages that they have communicated and help them create goals based on what they've said. You can ask your patients to summarize what they have learned from their session with you and what they plan to do once they leave. Use this information to help tailor your message to your patients' specific needs. Whenever Wendy does this, her patients happily respond after they jokingly ask why they have to pay her if they are the ones doing all of the work.

Tom: I know you want me to exercise, but I just can't do it. I really hate all forms of exercise. I think it is such a waste of time. I would much rather be sitting on the couch watching other people move!

You: You really feel strongly about not exercising. You think it is a poor use of your time and prefer to do something less strenuous. Is that right? (*Reflecting his comments.*)

Tom: Yes. You got that right! (*He feels heard.*)

You: Was there ever a time when you did enjoy exercising?

Tom: I used to be on a sports team. I really enjoyed running around with friends, loved scoring, and felt so young and flexible.

You: Ok, let me *summarize* what you've said so far. You actually do like exercising when you aren't alone. You enjoy the camaraderie of being part of a team. That is something to explore. So, let's shift our focus from "exercise" to "physical activity." Can you think of a way to increase your level of physical activity? Could you see this as something you could do for yourself?

Support Groups

Many patients benefit from learning in the presence of others who have similar medical issues. They learn that they are not alone, share solutions, and enjoy support. Compile a list of support groups in your geographic area you can share with your patients. Include different types of groups on your list, not only diabetes-related ones. Our patients often need help with eating disorders, addictions, and smoking cessation. If you struggle to change certain behaviors, follow your patients' lead and attend or start a colleague-based support group for yourself.

Tell Me More

Be inquisitive and curious. Don't jump to judgment. When patients bring up an issue, ask how they see the problem. This not only helps your patients feel that you value their opinions, it also improves your connection with them. Tell Me More also provides you with valuable information that can help keep you from working too hard to persuade your patients to do something they aren't ready to do. It also can help calm things down when a patient criticizes you. If a patient says, "I did what you said and it didn't work!" Your blood may start to boil, but don't act on that. First, SDR and then say, "Tell me more." Your patient's difficulty with your directive may have nothing to do with you or may be the result of a miscommunication.

Time Out

We can't eliminate all stresses from our lives, but we can become more adept at handling these stresses if we take a break whenever we feel overwhelmed. If you just finished arguing with an insurance representative or are angry about some news you received, take a few minutes to breathe and stretch to calm yourself down (APA, n.d.). Encourage your patients to do the same. If they become emotional during a session, gently tell them to take a moment and breathe while you step out of the room for 5 minutes. Not only will this help them focus better when you return, but also they will have learned an effective way to handle stress anytime, anywhere.

Visualization

If you are a fan of the Olympics, you may have noticed that many of the athletes close their eyes and run through their routine in their heads before they compete. They are using visualization, a mental technique that enables us to watch ourselves attempt a challenge and achieve a desired goal. You and your patients don't have to be sports competitors to use it. You can visualize yourself asking your boss for additional time off and getting it. Your patients can visualize themselves checking their blood and being pleased when their numbers appear on their glucose meter, regardless of the result. Research shows that "mental practices are almost as effective as true physical practice, and that doing both is more effective than either alone" (Le Van, 2009). To be effective, try to make the visualization as real as possible. In the case of glucose meter fears, encourage your patients to mentally walk themselves through as many details of their test as possible. Have them close their eyes and watch themselves enter their home, smell dinner cooking on the stove, pull up a chair at their dining room table (or wherever they test), feel the weight of the meter, open it up, pull it out, set it down, open up the strip bottle, and so on. Visualization, according to Le Van (2009) helps "enhance motivation, increase confidence and self-efficacy, improve motor performance, [and] prime your brain for success."

What Went Well

At the start of every appointment, ask your patients: "What went well since we last met?" This strength-based question helps you and your patients see the growth they have made. You can build on these strengths:

You: Hi, Dave, *what went well* since we saw each other 3 months ago?

Dave: I started eating a healthier breakfast. Lunch and dinner are still a disaster, but breakfast is really good.

You: I'm really impressed. A healthy breakfast is a great way to start your day, and you are doing that. I see that your post-breakfast blood glucose results reflect that as well. Are you ready to start to try another step?

Dave: Yeah. Let's take a look at lunch.

We are always too quick to focus on everything that is wrong. When you focus on what has improved and what is going well, you help enhance your patients' confidence, which can help them continue to make healthy choices and more effectively address things in their lives that may not be going as smoothly. Focus on the positive in your personal and professional life and see what happens. See how many things really go well for you each day.

The Takeaway

Face strong emotions (yours and your patients'). Use these approaches in all areas of your life, including at home and at work.

6
Emotions: Yours, Mine, and Ours

In this chapter, you will learn the following:

- Common emotions you or your patients may experience
- How these emotions can affect interactions
- Suggested actions you can take

Your "Next-Time" Guide

The following is a brief overview of some common emotions you may observe or feel during a patient session. We are highlighting these to help you develop "emotional literacy"—that is, to recognize, empathize, understand, and competently handle and respond to feelings you display and are displayed by others (Goleman, 1997). Beneath each entry, we offer some suggested actions from Chapters 4 and 5 that you can use to return the focus of your session back to your collaborative goals. Think of the following list as a quick "next-time" guide. You may not be prepared to address particular emotions when they show up the first time, but you can look them up here and choose what to try the next time they appear.

The actions we suggest beneath each emotion are exactly that—suggestions. Use any approach from Chapters 4 or 5 that you believe may be helpful, including one or more of your own. Don't be afraid of these emotions, address them head on. Many are a normal part of living with a chronic disease, so we need to know how to negotiate them. Just be sure to first tackle your own feelings using the stop, drop, and roll (SDR) intervention. Follow with "naming" to identify the emotion then "affirm" that this feeling is common, before you attempt an additional approach. Utilize the expertise of your behavioral health colleague to follow up as needed.

Your "Next-Time" List
Anger (Resentment)

> *No man can think clearly when his fists are clenched.*
> —George Jean Nathan

It isn't easy to interact with a patient who is angry or to assist someone while you feel this strong emotion. Your patients may feel angry about their diagnosis, the challenges that come with this disease, loved ones who nag them, or even at themselves for not tending to their personal health needs. While meeting with you, they may focus their anger on you, become cynical, criticize you, and reject your help. In the past, U.S. culture discouraged people from outwardly displaying anger, which is why many never learn to deal with this emotion in a constructive way (APA, 2013). Sadly, television reality shows now glorify aggressive displays when they feature brawling celebrities and screaming stage mothers.

For some people, anger is a habitual response. You probably know people who are constantly angry at almost everyone and everything in their lives. It's as if anger is their sole default emotion. Anger does have a positive side, however. It provides us with valuable feedback about ourselves when it highlights something that needs to be changed. If we dig deeper and search for the underlying source of our anger, we are likely to identify unmet expectations (past or present) we have of ourselves or of others (Allan, 2005). Patients who are angry about their poor diabetes control can use this strong emotion to prompt themselves to achieve their self-care health goals. Anger ignites change, passivity doesn't.

We may become angry when our patients ignore our guidance. According to Harville Hendrix, one of the founders of Imago Couples' Therapy, we don't have to agree with someone who feels angry, but it is "incumbent upon us to understand from their point of view why they are so angry or upset or resistant"

(Hendrix, 2008). Hopefully, when that happens, everyone involved will feel a greater sense of calm. Many individuals must feel that they are understood before they attempt to make any changes.

We, as well as our patients, also can bring anger from a previous event into the exam room. If you have a difficult phone call to make, hold off until you complete your appointments or at least until you feel calm enough to handle the conversation with aplomb. We can SDR and use other approaches to help keep our momentary anger from negatively affecting our judgment and our relationships with patients, colleagues, and loved ones. Allan (2005) suggests a quick mental exercise that can help you drop your anger when you SDR: Replace the expletive four-letter word that is racing around in your mind with a four-letter word that represents the unfulfilled source of your anger, such as "need," "goal," or "want."

Consider trying the following techniques: SDR and naming; anticipate, assertive language; collaborative conversation; deep breathing; feelings pass; listen, empathize, affirm, and positively reframe (LEAP); letter writing and journaling; referral to a behavioral health specialist; self-talk; slow down; summarizing; know your history; time out; what went well (WWW); and other options of your choice.

Anxiety (Worry)

If you or your patients feel anxious, try to see this as a helpful reminder that communicates the need to change a behavior or attitude. Diabetes self-care demands can be overwhelming. We and our patients fear possible complications, the cost, and other concerns. In addition to these stresses, some of your patients may be anxious about the goals they set. Note any sudden weight gain or erratic blood glucose results as your patients may eat to soothe their anxiety or calm the worry that they might have a future hypoglycemic or hyperglycemic event. Anxiety can be caused by biochemical issues, past experiences, stressful relationships, and other problems not directly related to diabetes.

Some of the physical symptoms of anxiety resemble those of hypoglycemia or a rapid drop in blood glucose, so encourage your patients to check their blood to make certain that they aren't experiencing a glucose low that requires treatment. Chronic symptoms include sleeping difficulties, shortness of breath, a racing heart, sweating, dizziness, and blood pressure changes. An actual low blood glucose level, or the fear of having one, also can prompt increased feelings of anxiety (McCoy, 2013).

Some patients and professionals respond to new technology with excitement and renewed motivation, whereas others feel overwhelmed. In today's medical environment, many health care providers become anxious when they are pushed to see a greater number of patients in less time. According to Lang (2005), when we warn our anxious patients about potential pain or attempt to be sympathetic while they go through a painful event, they may feel an even greater level of anxiety. As Wendy, one of our authors has observed, some patients do feel more relieved when they walk through the experience ahead of time as it helps desensitize the event.

Consider trying the following techniques: SDR and naming; anticipate, collaborative conversation; deep breathing; education; externalizing conversation; LEAP; mindfulness; referral to a behavioral health specialist; reprioritizing; role-play; scaling; searching for exceptions; slowing down; asking strength-based questions; tell me more; WWW; and options of your choice.

Defensiveness

People can become defensive if they feel attacked or dismissed. Our patients and their family members can feel this way when the information they share, actions they take, or advice they follow is belittled by their health care provider as being ineffective or foolish. Our patients may become defensive when relatives criticize or try to participate in their self-care decisions. No words have to be exchanged—a roll of the eyes, a gasp of surprise, or an awkward moment of silence can communicate disapproval.

We can feel defensive when patients or their family members share a medical perspective we don't endorse, seek a second opinion, or openly challenge our knowledge or decisions. We may also become defensive when our opinion is openly contradicted by our colleagues. The issue is not to suppress this feeling, but to respond in a way that strengthens the relationships we have with our patients and fellow staff members.

Consider trying the following techniques: SDR and naming; appreciation; collaborative conversation; deep breathing; education; externalizing conversation; LEAP; mindfulness; referral to a behavioral health specialist; reprioritizing; role-play; search for exceptions; self-compassion; tell me more; time out; WWW; and other options of your choice.

Denial

Denial can be healthy or unhealthy. As a healthy defense mechanism, it protects us from feeling frightened and anxious about stressful issues we are not ready to face. Consider the patient with type 2 diabetes (T2D) who denies his fear of needles so he can inject his insulin. Or the diabetes educator who pushes past her discomfort with technology so she can learn how to support her patients who wear insulin pumps. Once people establish healthy habits, it makes sense for them to experience denial about long-term diabetes-related complications. As long as they care for their health in a proactive way, they are less likely to develop these problems. In its unhealthy role, patients may ignore the value of a particular treatment when they incorrectly assume it is too late for their condition to improve.

Wendy originally coined the term "psychological insulin resistance" (Leslie, 1994). That's the unhealthy emotional barrier some patients and professionals erect, often mutually, against using insulin as a treatment option. When this occurs, patients may deny themselves the benefit of this medication because of the following concerns: They fear needles, feel like failures (if they see insulin as a punishment), worry about weight gain, feel it's too much hassle, fear that their diabetes has worsened, or are afraid of hypoglycemia (Davidson, 2012).

Patients also may deny themselves other beneficial treatment options if they don't recognize how capable they are of handling diabetes tasks or because, as with home glucose testing, they don't understand how to use the information. They also may deny the contribution their personal behavior makes to their medical issues, such as the patient who drinks copious amounts of sugar-sweetened beverages and then doesn't make the connection between his behavior and his poor diabetes control.

We may hesitate to prescribe a particular medication if we feel its use in certain patients represents a failure in our medical abilities. Our fear of failure can prompt us to deny the value of additional training, so we don't go for an advanced certification or degree. Most tragic is if we deny certain patients the benefit of the doubt and assume that they will never change because they showed no sign of change in the past.

Consider trying the following techniques: SDR and naming; education; empathic confrontation; gratitude; humor; LEAP; letter writing and journaling; referral to a behavioral health specialist; slow down; support groups; tell me more; visualization; and other options of your choice.

Depression and Diabetes-Related Distress

Depression and diabetes have a bidirectional relationship: People with diabetes have a greater risk of becoming clinically depressed and individuals who are depressed increase their risk of developing T2D (Pan, 2010). Evidence also suggests that "antidepressant use may be an independent risk factor for type 2 diabetes" (Barnard, 2013). As professionals, we sometimes feel depressed in response to certain situations, such as when patients develop complications or when they die. We also may feel depressed if we doubt the impact we have on our patients and their futures, or if we don't enjoy our current field of work.

When diabetes and depression are both present, people experience "increased functional impairment, more hospital days and days off of work, poorer glycemic control, poorer self-management behavior, increased health care use and costs, and a higher risk of morbidity and mortality" (Fisher, 2007). Note, however, that "most patients with diabetes and high levels of depressive symptoms are not clinically depressed" (Fisher, 2007). Instead, these individuals have diabetes-related distress, which is an "emotional response to a demanding health-related condition" (Fisher, 2014). According to Fisher (2014), one way to help patients deal with this issue is to utilize approaches that "include anticipating and acknowledging diabetes stressors over time, normalizing the experience of diabetes-related distress as part of the spectrum of diabetes, and recognizing how other life stressors can affect diabetes management." You can use several versions of the Problem Area in Diabetes Scale (PAID) to identify patients with diabetes-related distress. Two scales that are brief and psychometrically robust are PAID–1 and PAID–5. To learn more about diabetes-related distress, we recommend articles authored by Lawrence Fisher, PhD. Several of his titles are cited in the reference section of this book.

Consider trying the following techniques: SDR and naming; deep breathing; depression screening; externalizing conversation; journaling; LEAP; prayer; positive reframe; referral to a behavioral health specialist; self-compassion; self-disclosure, slow down; stories; WWW; and other options of your choice.

Embarrassment

Many of our patients feel too embarrassed to discuss topics of an intimate nature, such as sexual functioning. They may be embarrassed to share their blood glucose records with us if they believe the results show evidence of any poor diabetes care decisions, such as late-night overeating. We need to help our patients verbalize concerns that are on their minds. When they find the courage to open up, support them. While we may feel angry or upset by something they share, try not to show it or they will be less likely to reach out to us when future embarrassing issues arise.

We must find a way to overcome any personal awkwardness we may have with certain issues. We may have grown up with the notion that some topics should never be discussed or may worry that our age or gender doesn't give us the right to inquire about intimate subjects. Out of a group of 170 men, 82% stated that they wished their doctor had brought up the topic of erectile dysfunction (Baldwin, 2003). Our patients are counting on us to ask. If it helps, challenge yourself as Janis did in the following (originally shared in Marrero, 2008):

> After lecturing to many health care providers about the importance of discussing sexual complications with patients, Janis became keenly aware that she didn't do that with all of her own patients. So, she pledged to ask every patient she saw about his or her sexual performance, starting with her very next patient. To her surprise (and shock) her next patient was a Chassidic rabbi, complete with a long black coat, long beard and *peyot* (side curls). Her pledge suddenly seemed like a terrible idea! But she went ahead and mentioned to the rabbi that diabetes could affect a person's intimate life. Then she waited for his response. At first, he looked down at the floor and didn't utter a word. Janis became worried—was he offended? Did she overstep a boundary? Suddenly, the rabbi looked up and, in a very soft voice, admitted that he hadn't had sexual relations with his wife in more than 10 years. His disclosure opened up the discussion and Janis was able to provide important treatment and referral information.

Consider trying the following techniques: SDR and naming; affirm; cognitive restructuring; education; humor; LEAP; letter writing and journaling; referral to a behavioral health specialist; role-play (to help colleagues overcome their embarrassment); and other options of your choice.

Fear

Have you ever used fear to try to motivate your patients? Did you ever tell any of your patients that they would need insulin if they didn't take better care of themselves? It's not only unfair to categorize a health treatment as a punishment, it's inaccurate. For example, some patients require insulin regardless of how well they care for their health. Fear may prompt an initial behavior change, but it doesn't last long (Toll, 2010). This emotion, according to Dr. Judson Brewer, whom we quoted in our discussion about mindfulness, can prompt your patients "to *not* change behaviors." When some of Brewer's patients try to stop smoking, they cut way back, but they can't eliminate their final two or three cigarettes per day: "They are afraid of losing their identity, they don't know how to work with stress without smoking, they will lose their friends" (Brewer, 2013).

When patients enter the exam room feeling fearful, acknowledge their feelings. They may have a good reason to feel this way. Diabetes can be a frightening disease with very scary health and financial consequences. Your patients may not only fear diabetes complications, they also may believe they are inevitable. Listen and help calm their fears. That will bring better results than using their fear as a motivational tool. If your patients are afraid to attempt a certain task, ask them to break it into small steps so they can build up their comfort level slowly. If their fear comes from misinformation, invite them to share what they know about a particular topic so you can identify what might be upsetting them. Watch for fears that require a referral to the behavioral health professional on your team, such as an extreme fear of gaining weight or the frequent omission of insulin that could signal the presence of an eating disorder. Statements such as "After listening to you, I understand why you feel that way" or "We used to think that, but now we know" acknowledge patients beliefs so they don't feel you have dismissed them.

As professionals, we can get swept up in our patients' concerns and fear for them as well. According to Ofri (2013b), "Fear is woven into the daily existence of medicine—fear that we will harm our patients, kill them, forget something, [or] miss a diagnosis." We may worry that we aren't helping them as much as we believe we should be. We may fear that we won't be able to comfort our patients if and when they experience any change in their condition. Without acknowledging the presence of fear, this strong emotion can paralyze both us and our patients.

Consider trying the following techniques: SDR and naming; boundary setting; deep breathing; education; empathic confrontation; LEAP; letter writing and journaling; mindfulness; referral to a behavioral health specialist;

role-play; reprioritizing; self-talk; scaling; silence; slow down; visualization; and other options of your choice.

Frustration

It can be terribly frustrating when patients don't achieve their diabetes goals. Our patients can feel frustrated as well, especially if they want to please you or members of their family. Those who embrace challenges and see obstacles as tools that prompt growth can limit their frustration and become more resilient. Others, who don't welcome challenges and see obstacles as simply things that get in the way, will continue to struggle. These different mind-sets explain why some people stop reaching for goals and neglect to anticipate possible obstacles (Dweck, 2007). On the positive side, this emotion helps us identify individuals who have goals; you can't become frustrated if you don't set out to achieve something.

Think of what frustrates you: patient failures (not necessarily your fault), an inability to connect with some patients (again, not always your fault), repeat patient cancellations, lack of recognition from your peers, inadequate office support, or demands to see more patients in less time. You also may feel frustrated if you attempt to learn a new technology and fail to master it right away. When frustrated, you may make unreasonable demands of your patients, such as expecting them to do everything perfectly to manage their diabetes, which will only cause you and your patients to experience additional frustration.

Consider trying the following techniques: SDR and naming; education; encouraging; LEAP; letter writing and journaling; mindfulness; miracle question (abbreviated); network; reinforcing; referral to a behavioral health specialist; self-talk; slow down; support groups; time out; WWW; and other options of your choice.

Guilt and Shame

Feeling guilt or shame can prevent individuals from seeking the help they need. Shame occurs when people define themselves in a singular, negative way: "I am bad; I am a mistake." Guilt happens when one focuses on a thought or behavior and thinks, "I did something bad." According to Dr. Sanjay Gupta of CNN, people with diabetes carry an "extra burden of shame" (Gupta, 2013). This, he says, is because individuals who develop T2D "tend to be obese, and we still think of obesity as a self-created illness." Dr. Peter Attia, surgeon and co-founder of Nutrition Science Initiative, an organization that focuses on ways to lower "the individual, social, and economic costs associated with obesity-related diseases (Attia, 2012), admitted that his acceptance of this notion caused him to display less sympathy toward one of the patients with diabetes he encountered in an emergency room as a surgical resident. In an interesting twist of fate, Dr. Attia, who prided himself on exercising regularly and eating well, later developed T2D. He shares his personal story in the Ted-med talk, "Peter Attia: What if blaming the obese is blaming the victims?" (Tedmed, 2013). Wendy also observed that many people with type 1 diabetes feel shame as well. Having diabetes makes them feel different or "less than" others around them and prompts them to hide many of their self-care attempts from those who might criticize them.

To help yourself, your loved ones, and your patients move beyond the paralyzing feelings of guilt and shame, share insightful messages from Brené Brown's book, *The Gifts of Imperfection: Let Go of Who You Think You're Supposed to Be and Embrace Who You Are* (Brown, 2010). In it, she shares the value of changing our self-talk to help assuage what we feel: "You made a mistake. You're human. You're okay." She also encourages those who feel shame or guilt to tell their stories as a way to help process their feelings and move beyond them. We suggest you add, "I'm a good person who happens to have diabetes."

As a health care professional, you may feel guilty if you steal time from your busy practice to enjoy a relaxing lunch in your center's sunny courtyard. You might feel guilty if you discover that you have treated your co-workers or staff unfairly. Let's go easier on ourselves and our patients and use any guilt or shame we feel to motivate us all to grow and become our best selves.

Consider trying the following techniques: SDR and naming; appreciation; education; empathic confrontation; encouragement; feelings pass; forgiveness; LEAP; letter writing and journaling; miracle question; motivational interviewing; referral to a behavioral health specialist; silence; slow down; support groups, or other options of your choice.

Hate

Patients who hate their diagnosis and the behavior commitments that go with it may have a harder time engaging with you during an appointment. As with guilt, if channeled properly, your patients can use their intense feelings to motivate themselves to take steps that improve their health. Because hate often is rooted in unresolved issues from the past, it may be necessary to enlist a health behavioral professional to help your patients explore their anger, so they can move forward. If ignored, hate can move a person to become isolated and emotionally exhausted, especially if their hateful behaviors frighten themselves and others around them. As a health care professional, any hatred you feel toward your patients, workplace, significant other, or life in general can negatively affect your ability to do your job well. When you experience this emotion, view it as a valuable red flag that highlights something in your world that requires attention and must change.

Consider trying the following techniques: SDR and naming; LEAP; empathic confrontation; forgiveness; letter writing and journaling; mindful breathing; prayer; referral to a behavioral health specialist; silence; slow down; time out; and other options of your choice.

Hopelessness

It is reasonable for patients with diabetes to feel hopeless at some point in their lives, at least temporarily. After all, many patients have friends and family members who enthusiastically share horror stories of relatives with diabetes who died young or lost limbs. But their hopelessness can get in the way of hearing the hopeful and more accurate information you wish to share. Encourage your patients not to listen to frightening stories about people who were diagnosed more than 20 years ago, when the practice of diabetes care was far less advanced.

Hopelessness and depression tend to go hand in hand. Utilize the services of the health behavioral professional on your team if this emotion takes hold of you or any of your patients. Evidence suggests that feelings of hopelessness may be "important in the development and progression of [coronary heart disease]" (Dunn, 2014). Address these feelings promptly before medical issues develop that may become difficult to treat.

You can feel hopeless as a reaction to your own inability to master a new skill or when faced with mountains of administrative red tape, inconsiderate scheduling, and supervisors who marginalize your concerns. You also may feel hopeless as a reaction to a patient's newly developed complication or to his or her feeling of hopelessness.

Consider trying the following techniques: SDR or naming; depression screening; education; externalizing conversation; LEAP; referral to a behavioral health specialist; stories; support groups, and other options of your choice.

Hurt

Many of our patients feel hurt when loved ones don't support their diabetes self-care tasks in ways they would like them to. Some may feel so hurt that they ignore their diabetes needs because they fear they won't have adequate support to achieve their health goals. Patients also can feel hurt when we or members of our staff seem insensitive to their needs. Dutton (as quoted in Potera, 2010) asked 143 patients with a BMI of more than 25 kg/m^2 to list weight-loss terminology their physicians used that they found hurtful. None approved of the word "fatness," which was not surprising, but they listed the word "obesity" as being almost as hurtful. Patients also were not in favor of the terms "excess fat, large size, ... and heaviness." The word "weight" was deemed acceptable as were (in order of diminishing preference) "BMI, unhealthy body weight, unhealthy BMI, weight problem, and excess weight" (Dutton, as quoted in Potera, 2010) Always monitor your patients' reactions to the terminology you use to see whether any words cause distress. We are healers and educators. The last thing we want to do is hurt those we wish to help.

We may feel hurt by patients who don't listen to our advice, who are disappointed in us, or who criticize us. We also can feel hurt by colleagues and staff who we believe don't respect us as well as by administrators who ignore or minimize our requests.

Consider trying the following techniques: SDR or naming; empathic confrontation; externalizing conversation; LEAP; referral to a behavioral health specialist; slow down; support groups; role-play; self-talk; and other options of your choice.

Sadness

No one jumps for joy when they are diagnosed with diabetes, although they initially may feel relieved to learn that their troubling symptoms have a definitive cause. Our patients feel sad at times: They face an uncertain future and have a chronic illness that has no immediate cure, is misunderstood by the public as well as by others in their lives, requires daily attention, and can significantly strain one's finances. Patients can feel sad if they develop complications, learn about fellow patients who have succumbed to diabetes-related medical issues, have bosses who don't respect their health needs, or feel angry and have no healthy outlet in which they can express their feelings. Abnormal and fluctuating blood glucose levels can prompt sad feelings (Zrebiac, 2011), so encourage your patients to check their blood when they feel this emotion to verify that they don't have a blood glucose level that they need to treat. When children are diagnosed with diabetes, their parents experience numerous loss-related emotions, including sorrow. As time goes on, many parents adapt and cope, but some develop a "chronic sorrow" that continues for many years beyond their child's initial diagnosis (Lowes, 2000).

As health care providers, we can feel sad for a variety of reasons, including when we lose valued patients because they move away, pass away, see a different physician, or develop complications. Sometimes our patients' sadness will trigger this emotion in us, too. We or our patients also may feel sad because of personal issues, an inherited biochemical tendency, or even normal hormonal changes, such as menstrual periods and menopause. Certainly lack of sleep, changes in our workload or finances, or personal disappointments, such as marital stress, child-rearing challenges, and aging parents, can prompt us to feel sad.

Consider trying the following techniques: SDR or naming; depression screening; LEAP; feelings pass; letter writing and journaling; referral to a behavioral health specialist; slow down; stories; tell me more; WWW; and other options of your choice.

Stress

Patients who experience a great deal of stress in their lives, in addition to their diabetes, may be less likely to do all they need to improve their health. In the office, they may act indifferent or use most of the session to share how overwhelmed they feel. Stress can negatively affect blood glucose levels. For some patients, a high level of stress can prompt them to try to relieve the pressure by engaging in excessive drinking, eating, or drug use. If you are a professional who works in a stressful environment, your exhausting workload can cause you to lose sleep and make poor (and possibly dangerous) decisions.

On the other hand, stress can be a great motivator. We help our patients see it this way when we name their stress (don't ignore it) and positively reframe it as a challenge rather than a burden. McGonigal (2009) urges people to consider the "upside of stress" and see it as something that helps "create resilience." When we and our patients adopt this attitude, we can use stress to motivate us to greater success.

Consider trying the following techniques: SDR or naming; deep breathing; education; empathic confrontation; externalizing conversation; humor; LEAP; mindfulness; network; referral to a behavioral health specialist; reprioritizing; self-talk; slow down; and other options of your choice.

Lack of Motivation

People feel unmotivated when they don't see a reason to do a particular action or have failed to reach a goal after numerous attempts. They may feel less motivated if they are depressed or distressed about their diabetes. Some incorrectly attribute their lack of motivation to a *lack* of willpower, which is "the ability to resist short-term temptations in order to meet long-term goals" (APA, 2014). McGonigal, author of *The Willpower Instinct* (2011), states that willpower is a "biological function," not an abstract feeling. With training, she believes we can use mindfulness and heightened awareness of things that distract us to overcome negative impulses; to relax and reduce stress; and, in turn, to increase our willpower. According to Baumeister (2011), it isn't just a matter of "making up your mind." Willpower tends to be highest in the morning, so encourage your patients, as well as yourself, to attempt challenging changes earlier in the day.

Consider trying the following techniques: SDR or naming; affirm; education; empathic listening; mindfulness; encouragement; letter writing and journaling: referral to a behavioral health specialist; reprioritizing; strength-based questions; support groups; WWW; and other options of your choice.

The Takeaway

You and your patients can approach your emotions in new and more meaningful and effective ways.

7
It Takes a Village

Spoon feeding in the long run teaches us nothing but the shape of the spoon.
—Edward Morgan Forster

In this chapter, you will learn the following:

- How to utilize the strengths of group participants to enhance learning

In January 2005, Janis took a taxi from her hotel in Jerusalem to the nearby Yad Sarah center to speak at the monthly meeting of the lay division of the Israel Diabetes Association. Everything that could have gone wrong did. First, the weather—the rain that evening was so heavy that her shoes and dress became saturated as she dashed from the cab to the entrance of the building. The center only had an ancient laptop that couldn't run her slides. Additionally, the translator for the evening was running late due to heavy traffic. As awful as the evening should have been, it ended up being one of the highlights of Janis' career. That's because working with groups is not only about the information one shares, it is also about the connections that are made. Despite the language barrier, which could have turned this presentation into a noninteractive lecture, Janis communicated her warmth and affection to all who came that evening (the room was packed!), and the attendees shared their warmth and energy with her as well as with each other. Using her limited Hebrew, she engaged everyone in a discussion about diabetes eating challenges—what worked for them and what didn't. When the translator and replacement laptop finally arrived, Janis shared the rest of her presentation and ended the evening with a wonderfully interactive question–answer period.

If you lead diabetes education classes, you probably stand up in front of groups, present information, lead a meaningful question–answer period, and then say goodbye. If you have additional time, you may incorporate some creative hands-on experiences, use visual aids, or even invite attendees to participate in a few team exercises. All of these methods disseminate valuable information participants can use.

We'd like to help you take these interactions to the next level and enhance the communication and learning that goes on during each session. Ongoing support groups, single drop-in educational sessions, lectures, and even shared medical appointments (which are growing in popularity) can be more than simply cost-effective ways to get facts and resources to a larger number of people in a limited amount of time. If run well, they can provide opportunities for everyone present to communicate in ways that differ from face-to-face sessions. Participants not only can learn new skills but also can discuss their feelings, share their emotional responses to diabetes and its care tasks, teach others, develop supportive relationships, and begin to feel more hopeful and capable.

Those who attend are not the only ones who benefit from educational and supportive group gatherings. The professionals who run them gain as well. When we present a topic once to a group rather than multiple times in face-to-face sessions, we reduce our risk of becoming bored. Each group meeting gives us an opportunity to spend more time with the participants, so we can tackle more issues and develop more fulfilling bonds. We also learn from group members who participate in discussions and offer new ideas. We aren't standing alone. Members assist and support us and become part of our team. And groups are fun! Unfortunately, many people are either afraid to do this type of work or think they won't enjoy the experience. Wendy has taught group work at the University of Maine's Graduate School of Social Work for 22 years. Each semester, she sees students grow from timid to excited about running groups. If you don't feel ready to work with groups at this time, attend a few sessions that are run by colleagues to see what they do. You hopefully will enjoy what you see. If you feel so inclined, offer to assist the leader for the evening, so you can interact with group members without being totally in charge.

The following information deals with groups that are either ongoing or are part of programs that offer different sessions people can attend. If your group only meets a single time, a great deal of what we share will be very helpful. We hope you will read through the entire chapter and, as we tell those who attend the groups we run, take what has meaning for you!

Starting the Session

When you enter the room for the first time, set a tone of acceptance and under-standing. Smile. Introduce yourself and mention your credentials. The group members need to know they can rely on the accuracy of the information they will learn. Tell everyone how excited you are that they came, that you believe in their power to change their lives for the better, and that they can help their fellow group members do the same. If you are nervous, you can let them know. That admission will demonstrate your honesty and model how forthcoming you hope they will be.

People respond differently when they enter a group setting for the first time. Some are excited and look forward to connecting with others. They are ready to share, connect, and learn. Some feel anxious and are worried about how they may be judged. They don't know who you are, are afraid to speak in front of others, and may worry that you will tell them things that negatively affect their quality of life (i.e., no more chocolate, no more alcohol, etc.). They may worry that they will say something stupid or share too many personal details. Your empathetic, accepting, and welcoming attitude can help ease their discomfort.

Make Introductions

Go around the room and ask everyone to introduce themselves. This style of asking questions by going from person to person is known as a "round." Invite participants, one by one, to say their name and state a single brief piece of information, such as their best quality or what diabetes task they handle well. This round breaks the ice, gives everyone a chance to speak in front of fellow group members, and helps the group begin to focus on their strengths. Those who are hesitant will appreciate that you only want them to say a few brief words—they can get through it quickly. After everyone speaks, members, hopefully, will observe that everything said in the group does not have to be brilliant or worded perfectly. If one or more participants walk into the group late, don't ignore them and continue what you are doing. Stop for a moment, acknowledge their presence, and inform them of the topic, so they can join in the session. Smile and say, "Hi! Welcome! Please take a seat. I will have you introduce yourself in a few minutes. We are just talking about how to make healthy food choices when eating out (or another topic)." Then return to what you were doing. At the very next opportunity, begin another round in which everyone, including the newcomers, says their name and shares something brief, such as one reason why they decided to come.

It is great to start every session with a round. If your group meets again, have everyone say one thing that went well since you last met (what went well—WWW). Let them know that what they share can be quite small—perhaps they went to bed on time one night that week or thought about attending an aerobics class. Thinking about making a change is a positive step. The goal is to help your patients strengthen their feelings of competency (self-efficacy) and identify successes, regardless of how insignificant they may seem to be.

You can invite group members to suggest something to talk about at this meeting. Write their suggestions down on a white board and weave the topics into the discussion or set aside time at the end to discuss them. Some members may feel pressured by rounds (especially those who are more introverted). To ease this discomfort, have everyone first take out a pen and paper and jot down what they'd like to share. Also, give everyone permission to opt out and pass their turn to the next person. Rounds are especially helpful when a group lacks energy and focus. If you don't have a specific question ready, take a topic from the worksheets in Chapter 2.

Review the Rules

Rules put people at ease. Discuss the rules for the session and ask for the group's agreement. Be sure to include the following:

- Participants are invited to speak, but they also are welcome to stay silent.
- Everyone must respect, listen, and not judge fellow group members.
- All shared personal information is confidential—what happens in the group, stays in the group!

Once the rules are set, *enforce them*. Stop the session, if needed, to remind everyone of the rules they all agreed to follow. Appreciate that those who interrupt others may be excited to show what they know (*positive reframe*).

If they do interrupt, you and other members of the group should respectfully ask them to wait. Assure everyone that they all will have an opportunity to participate in the discussions.

In the next chapter, we will discuss introverted and extroverted individuals and how they may respond in certain situations. Many people don't like to speak up. Some are influenced by cultures that do not value self-disclosure, such as select members of the Asian American population, who might "learn emotional restraint at an early age and are expected to exhibit modesty in the face of authority as well as subtleness in dealing with personal problems" (Diller, 2007). These patients do their best learning by observing others or may need a little more time to review their thoughts before they choose to share them. Be cognizant and respectful of that. Connect with them through eye contact and smiles. But don't give up on them: They may begin to participate as their comfort level grows. Offer opportunities for all to speak. Don't assume that anyone who refuses to speak once will refuse again in the future.

Role-Play

We discussed the value of role-play in Chapter 5. In a group, you have a wonderful opportunity to use this approach. Don't simply talk about situations, choose members to act them out and experiment with different ways to approach each problem. For example, if one member worries about what to eat at a company holiday party, role-play the conversation between him and his co-worker. Have others suggest possible ways for the scenario to proceed. What happens if he turns down the doughnut that his co-workers offer, but they won't take no for an answer? What if other co-workers join the conversation and tease him about his food preferences? By acting out a scenario in multiple ways, the group gets an opportunity to help answer, "What if?" in a safe, supportive environment. Hopefully, the member with the issue will feel better able to handle the real-life situation. Remind all participants that they never will be alone because they always can "visualize" their supportive, fellow group members standing behind them. Another bonus of role-play is that it infuses some humor into the session. Humor acts as a social lubricant that relaxes people, promotes skill building, and helps group members bond and support one another (Rapaport, 2013).

Messages to Share

Groups offer participants an opportunity to express themselves and heighten their self-awareness. Don't lecture, but encourage members to share their thoughts. Maximize the power of each session by emphasizing the following (Yalom, 2005):

- Offer hope
- Affirm
- Celebrate altruism—the health benefits of helping others
- Be a healthier authority figure and provide opportunities for members to lead as well
- Model more successful social behaviors and coping strategies

Offer Hope

Everyone who lives with diabetes, from the newly diagnosed to the seasoned "old-timer," experiences daily ups and downs, physical and financial worries, and family stresses. All gain from messages of hope. Whenever your group meets, regardless of its purpose, infuse the session with realistic messages of hope that come from you and other members. Feeling hopeful helps patients return for future sessions. Let them know that what they learn can help them live better lives.

Affirm

As we've suggested throughout this book, people benefit when someone validates their feelings and lets them know that others have similar issues and concerns. According to Yalom (2005), "the disconfirmation of a client's feelings of uniqueness is a powerful source of relief." Share this powerful message with your group and encourage them to validate each other's feelings as well.

Celebrate Altruism

Several years ago, Janis gave a lecture at an American Association of Diabetes Educators' conference on how to raise patients' "Diabetes Self-Esteem." Asking patients to share in a group session is one way to do that. When members of your group help each other solve problems, their self-esteem rises as they develop their feelings of mastery over their diabetes and as they help others. During your group class or session, invite attendees to respond to questions that others pose. Don't stand at the front of the room and give out all the answers. Don't lecture. That is not only mentally exhausting, but it also denies your members an opportunity to grow. Turn as many questions back to the group as possible. When Kim asks, "How can I fit more walking into my day?" don't immediately respond with tips on how to use a pedometer. Toss the topic over to the group as you highlight that it was Kim's contribution to the discussion: "Kim, that's a good question for us to think about. How would all of you answer it?" Give the members of the group an opportunity to help one another. You might be surprised at the creative and helpful responses they give, so be sure to take notes.

Be a Healthier Authority Figure

You are an authority on diabetes. For some members of your group, the suggestions you offer may remind them of orders their parents or other early authority figures used to give. If they had a poor relationship with their parents, they may respond negatively when asked to participate in the group. React to their response in a healthy and appropriate way and encourage their fellow group members to respond positively as well. Help them explore the best way to use the information you discuss to manage their diabetes better.

Debbie, the diabetes educator, explained to her group how important it is to check their feet every day. Tom, one of the group members, mumbled, "Yeah, right. Another thing to add to my day. This is getting ridiculous!" Tom challenged Debbie and the demands of diabetes, just as he challenged his parents, teachers, and other authority figures who probably became angry when he reacted in such a contrary way. Today, Debbie has an opportunity to demonstrate a more positive response. But before she responds, she must first take care of her feelings. She feels angry because Tom challenged her recommendation. She uses the stop, drop, and roll (SDR) intervention to help assume a more compassionate and understanding attitude toward him and then she uses LEAP:

1. Listen
2. Empathize
3. Affirm
4. Positively reframe

Debbie: "Hi Tom. I heard what you said. (*Listen.*) It sounds like you are tired of all of the things you need to do to take care of your diabetes each day." (*Empathize and look around the room to see if others are nodding in agreement. If they are, point this out to Tom.*)

Tom: "I hate all of this! I can't believe that I now have to add 'check your feet' to the list. I hate having diabetes!"

Debbie: "You hate having diabetes and all of the things you have to do to take care of it. Lots of people feel that way some of the time. (*Affirm.*) Checking your feet doesn't have to take very long. I know one couple who checks each other's feet as part of a loving foot massage. (*Positively reframe.*)

Debbie involves the rest of the group by asking:

- How many of you have ever felt like Tom and how did you handle it?
- Do any of you also struggle with the same feelings? (Give members a chance to be altruistic and show Tom he is not alone.)
- Have any of you thought of ways to fit foot inspections into your day?
- Who has a suggestion for Tom?
- Would any of you like to try one of these suggestions at home?

Model More Successful Social Behaviors and Coping Strategies

Diabetes can negatively affect how many people socialize and interact with others (Holt, 2013). When people come to your group, you have an opportunity to reinforce appropriate social behaviors that participants can use with others. You also can help others identify positive strategies and behaviors that fellow members of the group already do. These behaviors include listening, not interrupting, making eye contact, showing appreciation and support, clarifying their preferences, giving honest compliments, and more. When you ignore certain behaviors because they seem too awkward or difficult to correct, you give them tacit approval. When one member interrupts another, acknowledge how enthusiastic they are to share, but remind them and the rest of the group that everyone must be quiet and respectful until their fellow members complete their comments. Again, you are not only an educator, you also teach by example. You respect everyone and don't shame others. And your group members can teach each other by modeling positive behaviors during sessions.

Getting Personal

Get the group's permission before you ask participants to share personal experiences. It shows you respect them and only want them to participate if they feel ready. Once you obtain their permission, ask how they personally deal with a specific health problem. Ask if others have ever had a similar experience. If you bring up a particularly uncomfortable topic, such as how their sex lives have changed, stop for a moment and listen to how your group reacts. Some may react strongly and criticize you for bringing up the topic. Don't let that upset you. SDR and then identify what you see—a group that is comfortable sharing their thoughts and is helping you see aspects of a topic that don't normally come to mind. Let the group know that this is a safe place to bring up troubling issues. If they want to criticize you, they can do that as well, as long as it is done in a positive way. Encourage them to share their thoughts and let you know if you are covering anything too rapidly. You may be tempted to share a personal story during a session. As we suggested earlier, experts differ on whether or not this is appropriate. Before you share something from your life, consider how it might be received by the group.

Prepare for Silence

At times, the group may not respond to a question you ask. Or you may see someone put his or her head down and look disinterested. Don't get nervous and break into a quick soft shoe or stand-up comedy routine. Silence, by a group or individual, often indicates that participants are thinking more deeply about an issue that you or someone else brought up (*positive reframe*). Keep smiling and wait or ask, "What are you thinking?" If you mentioned bike riding, for example, some of the people may take a moment to think how they can fit a nice bike ride into their week. They even may begin to daydream about how nice it would be to invite a friend to join them. These internal thoughts help them process what you said and make it real for them.

How to Handle Disruptions

If any participants dominate the conversation, handle the situation with compassion. They may have needs that they aren't verbalizing in an appropriate way. They may wish to help you out, compete with you, get attention, or even assist the other members of the group. They may act this way because they are trying to feel better about having diabetes, which currently makes them feel awful. If you don't encourage them to curb their negative behavior, however, other members may begin to dislike them and cringe every time they open their mouths to speak. When is the right time to deal with this type of situation? Monitor your own reactions. If you think this person dominates the conversation, others do too. Don't stay silent. Others in the group are looking to you to handle the situation, so they can feel comfortable and safe once again. When someone dominates, say, "I know you are interested in sharing and helping others. You always contribute with such great energy. We'll come back to you when everyone has had a chance to talk" or "Thank you for your comments, Susan. Anyone else?" Employ your nonverbal skills to encourage others to speak up. Shift your body toward a member who hasn't contributed yet. Look over at someone and use your eyes to invite him or her to share. If certain individuals continue to disrupt the session, meet with them afterward and encourage them to see an educator, one-on-one, instead of or in addition to their group sessions.

If members of the group criticize you, first SDR to calm your feelings and then say the following: "I'm so glad you told me how you feel" or "It took a lot of courage to say that. Thank you." You can also say, "That's interesting" or "Tell me more" (see Chapter 5). If they have numerous comments, devote time at the next session to hear their concerns, so everyone can work together to develop a more mutually satisfying way to run the group. If a single individual appears disgruntled, invite him or her to stay after for a few minutes or come early to the next session so you can devote more time to his or her concerns. When you do meet, ask this person to reflect back on what he or she says and compile a list of his or her suggestions. Use them to develop future sessions. If "Doris" criticizes you and other members rush to your defense, say, "It's so nice that you want to defend me. I feel it's fine that Doris shared her thoughts about how I run the group. I appreciate the fact that she felt comfortable enough to give me some constructive criticism. Offering and receiving helpful feedback can help us all improve."

What Would You Do?

Following are several scenarios that might come up in groups that you run. Read them through and think about how you would handle them. If a similar situation arises, use your own response, or feel free to try the ones we suggest.

Scenario 1

Sara, whose type 1 diabetes is poorly controlled, got up the courage to admit that she never checks her blood before she gets behind the wheel of a car. Sid, another member of the group, judges her harshly and whispers (loudly) to those near him that he thinks Sarah's behavior incredibly irresponsible! What should you do?

Our response: If you don't address his comment, Sara may be less likely to share future personal thoughts. Turn to Sid and point out that he obviously wants Sarah to behave in a different way for her safety and for the safety of others. (*Positive reframe.*) Ask him if he would tell her that same important comment again, but in a more supportive way. Remind him that we are all here to learn and support one another. It took a lot of courage for Sara to share this, and you appreciate that it also took courage for him to share his criticism. You want to make sure that she and everyone else continues to feel comfortable discussing personal stories. Thank them both for their contributions and invite Sid to share anything about Sara's comment that impressed him.

Scenario 2

Roger is a 65-year-old member of your beginner insulin pump class. He struggled all evening with his pump and kept pointing out how easy it was for everyone else in the room. "I feel so dumb. I just feel so dumb!" He stated over and over again. Finally, he stood up and yelled, "You are going too fast! I quit! I just can't do this anymore." What do you do?

Our response: First, SDR to deal with your own feelings. Roger just insulted your teaching style and that stings a bit. As you SDR, consider that Roger may have shared what others are feeling: You may be going through the material too quickly. That realization helps you see him in a more compassionate way. After you SDR, you LEAP: "Thank you, Roger, for telling us how frustrated you are. Maybe other members of the group need more time also. Can you talk more about what is upsetting you?" (*Listen.*) He tells you that the pump is too hard for him. He says that he is angry because he is too old to learn. You say, "Thank you for being so honest. It must feel awful to want to learn the pump so badly then find it hard to do." (*Empathize.*) You let him know that many people have a hard time at first. (*Affirm.*) Then suggest that his need to go more slowly shows how careful he is and that his attention to detail will help him have greater success when he finally begins to wear a pump.

(*Positive reframe.*) He begins to smile. You let him know that many people learn at a slower pace because they are so meticulous. Since he mentioned that he thinks he is too old for pumping, you share that numerous people his age are successful pump users, some even older than 70 years old (Roszler, 2002). Let him know how grateful you are for reminding you to mention that, if needed, everyone can meet with a private pump trainer in addition to or in place of the group session. You ask if he would like to meet with a pump trainer for private sessions, so he can learn at his own pace. He agrees and you tell him that you will help him make the arrangements. You turn to the group and share that it is courageous to voice our needs and struggles. "Roger, thank you for modeling this behavior for the rest of us." Follow this by inviting other members to share (in a single sentence) their reactions to Roger's concern and what they gained from hearing what he had to say.

Scenario #3

Nick refuses to answer any of your questions and just sits with his head on the table. What would you do?

Our response: Try to find out what is happening with Nick. Don't assume anything. You ask, "Nick, what's going on?" He says that he doesn't want to be there. (*Listen.*) You say that it must be hard to sit there when he really wishes he were somewhere else. (*Empathize.*) You thank him for letting you know how he feels and ask if there is something he would like to learn or discuss. He says that he would really like to know how to adjust his insulin so he can play sports with his friends. Tell him that this is a great topic for everyone in the group (*Affirm*) and let him know that his ability to identify and express his feelings so clearly shows a high level of self-awareness. (*Positively reframe.*) Then ask if he'd like to help you discuss it at the next session. He responds enthusiastically and says that he is excited about doing that. Nick feels heard and begins to pay more attention as the session continues. Again, throw this topic back to the group: Go around and ask everyone to briefly share what they gained from what they just observed.

Scenario #4

In the middle of a discussion about how diabetes affects your group members' personal relationships, Vicky suddenly tears up and starts to rummage through her purse to find a tissue. What do you do?

Our response: Like Vicky, some of your group participants are likely to become overwhelmed with sadness when certain topics arise. Don't ignore Vicky's feelings. Don't continue to talk or try to switch topics. Vicky needs to share her feelings and you are the one to help her do that. You also may not be the only one who sees her. Other group members who notice her can be moved by her strong emotions and want her to feel relief. Ask Vicky if she is willing or able to describe what she feels. Listen to her response. (*Listen.*) She says that she is upset because her diabetes is ruining her marriage. You say, "That must be so hard to live with a disease and have it affect your relationship with your husband so intensely." (*Empathize.*) Let her know that others in the group might be struggling with this also as it is a common problem that you've seen often. (*Affirm.*) Her comment also shows how much she values her marriage. (*Positive reframe.*) She says that she doesn't know if she is ready to share. You thank her for making everyone aware of an important situation others may want to discuss and for speaking up for those who may be less comfortable to do so. Encourage her to take her time and only talk when she feels ready.

Ending the Session

Wendy tells a story about the time she ended the final session of a six-session series for mothers whose children had diabetes: "I was ending our final session with my usual WWW and asked, "What have you gained from coming?" One mother opened up and said, "I love this group. You know I'm crazy about you, Wendy. I learned so many ways to handle difficult situations with my kids, their teachers, other relatives and friends. There is just one thing you missed—diabetes is really sad and difficult. I feel like you never gave us time to look at our sadness and anger."

When Wendy heard this, her heart sank. The mother was right. Wendy, who tends to be very upbeat, neglected to invite the mothers to explore the darker side of their diabetes-related emotions. "It was a pivotal moment for me," admitted Wendy. "This woman's feedback taught me something important. I looked around the room and raised my hand to stop the other mothers who wanted to defend me then turned back to that mother and said, 'I am so impressed with the kind and honest way that you said that to me. It doesn't matter if others feel differently. You do, and that's means a lot to me.'" In future sessions, Wendy made sure that she brought up more uncomfortable topics and ended every group series by not only asking WWW, but also WWNW (what went *not* so well!). Another way to end a session is to have everyone identify something they will do differently to manage their diabetes. This makes it more concrete and works to improve outcomes. Change isn't easy for anyone, including health care professionals who always are learning new things that benefit themselves as well as their patients.

As your session gets close to its ending time, set aside some time for everyone to share what they gained from the session and what they plan to do differently to help manage their diabetes. If this is the first in a series of meetings, ask the participants WWW. This question helps them think more positively. Ask what they enjoyed about the session and what they would like to change. Don't take their comments as criticism, but rather as a way for them to show their preferences. They may want more discussion time and less teaching or vice versa. Their comments show that they are aware of their needs. Before everyone departs, let them know how they can reach you if they have any comments or questions before the next session.

Logistics

Where your group meets communicates a great deal to your participants. It isn't a simple matter of logistics. Two years ago, Janis took over an established support group for divorced women (not diabetes related). At that time, the group met in a poorly lit library filled with dusty books. The room was down the hall from a classroom where some of the women's ex-husbands attended lectures. The women characterized their past sessions as "pity parties," in which everyone complained, moaned, and groaned. Janis quickly moved the group's location to a brightly lit conference room in a different building, several blocks from its original spot. The change was palpable. The members immediately became more animated and open about their concerns, shared advice, and began to feel more positive about their personal situations. If your group room is near a noisy cafeteria, in a poorly lit or chilly room, or has other negative aspects, address these issues or move to a better location.

A Matter of Size

The size of your group can enhance or hinder communication. If a group has three or fewer members, you may start to focus on individual issues and not develop the dynamic that is so unique to groups. The participants will have fewer opportunities to experience the "hall of mirrors effect" in which they see "multiple aspects of [themselves] reflected in other people" (Zrebiec, 2003). If your group is too large, it makes it harder for everyone to participate. A great starting number is 10–12 members. Assume that over time some participants will drop out or attend inconsistently. When that happens, your group will still be a workable size.

A Matter of Timing

The length of each session can either support communication or stifle it. Make it long enough to accomplish your goals and give members time to share. Don't go for so long that you exhaust yourself and the participants. If you limit the length of the session too much, members may be afraid to bring up more pressing topics because they take longer to discuss. Always start on time and end on time, so members don't leave while others are still speaking or feel that they are missing out on something valuable. If someone brings up an important issue toward the end of a session, it is tempting to continue for just a bit longer. Don't. Affirm the importance of the topic and assure the person who brought it to your attention that you will cover it in the next session. Between session, people often think about what they learned and come up with questions and concerns. At the following meeting, after you have everyone go around and share WWW, ask whether anyone has any lingering questions from the previous meeting. You also can add those questions to the evening's agenda.

Taking Over an Established Group

If you take over a group from a colleague, you will have to develop relationships with folks who may be very upset that their beloved "leader" is gone. Before you go it alone, attend one of the outgoing facilitator's final sessions, so he or she can introduce you to the group. That gives you his or her official approval, which will help the members accept you. When you run your first session, ask WWW? What went well in the past that the group members would like you to continue? Apply some of their suggestions to help smooth the transition. You can either keep these activities or gradually drop those that don't fit your style or philosophy. Make changes slowly or you are likely to run into resistance. If members quote the other leader: "Julie always did it *this* way" or "You say no, but Dave told us that it was okay to do that." First, SDR, so you keep your personal emotions in check and then validate their feelings. Let them know that you are impressed that they gained so much from past sessions. Some of the members may be angry that their other leader left, so give them an opportunity to share their thoughts. Let them know that you understand their anger because it is normal to be upset when a leader you cared about leaves (*affirm*). You may have a different perspective on some things, but you respect what the other leader shared with them and hope they will feel comfortable sharing additional information in the future. If you handle the transition well, they will grow to like and respect you and even may end up liking you more than the other leader.

Remember, you are going to facilitate the group, not lecture or entertain. *The group is the star, not you.* This "group-focused" perspective may be new for you. We hope you will give it a try. It requires that you step back, which may feel odd at first, especially if you like to have total control, but the potential for growth by your patients and by you can be quite impressive when you do step back. Don't worry, you are still in control, but you are allowing your group members to do most of the work. If you facilitate an ongoing support or educational group, we encourage you to learn more about the psychodynamics of group processes in greater depth. One book that is especially helpful is *The Theory and Practice of Group Psychotherapy* by Irvin D. Yalom (2005).

The Takeaway

Don't be afraid of groups: Members grow when they do most of the work.

8
Singing Kumbaya

n this chapter, you will learn the following:

- How to improve your workplace interaction style
- How to influence others to do their best work (even when you're not in charge!)

Most of us spend more time with co-workers than we do with our family and friends. For many of us, our co-workers *are* our family. So, in addition to the interactional approaches and group communication concepts we've already shared, we'd like to present a few more options that can help you expand your level of self-awareness and enhance your professional relationships.

Stop Molehills From Becoming Mountains

It isn't always possible to get along with everyone, every day at work. At some point, you or one of your co-workers is likely to say or do something that strains your relationship. Shari Harley, author of *How to Say Anything to Anyone: A Guide to Building Business Relationships That Really Work* (2013), encourages you to avoid major conflicts by inviting co-workers to support a critical ground rule, which is to be honest and open with you and vice versa. Here is how Harley (2013) suggests you introduce the idea:

I want a good relationship with you. If we work together long enough, I'm sure I'll screw it up. I'll wait too long to reply to an email, make a mistake, or miss a deadline. I'd like the kind of relationship in which we can always talk about these things. I always want to know what you think. And I promise that no matter what you tell me, I'll say thank you. Is it okay if I work this way with you?

You may word your invitation differently, but the message should be clear: You want to know of any concerns, *before* they get out of hand. If your co-workers agree, reconfirm this "agreement" every so often to ensure that you continue to interact at this level of openness.

Don Your Superhero Cape

Another way to set the stage for quality workplace interactions is to bring your most confident self to each conversation. A team led by social psychologist Amy Cuddy, associate professor at Harvard Business School, examined several physical stances and how they affected different individuals' confidence levels. Certain physical poses significantly altered their hormone balance, which affected their attitudes. According to Cuddy, most successful leaders have a high testosterone and low cortisol level, which allows them to be less defensive and better decision makers (Buchanan, 2012). It also increases their feeling of personal power and tolerance for risk (Carney, 2010; Peterson, 2012).

To improve your hormone balance, stand in a power pose for a minute or two. A power pose is a stance in which you extend your body and limbs. To do this, lift your arms high into the air as you walk around a room. Or, raise your hands up high as you stand up on your tiptoes. You can also stand, looking forward, with your legs apart and arms akimbo—the favored stance of Wonder Woman (the superhero outfit is optional!). In the study, subjects who stood for 1 minute in a power pose experienced a testosterone increase of 19% and a cortisol level drop of 25%. Their heightened feelings of confidence lasted approximately 15–30 minutes. On the other hand, those who assume a weaker pose experienced the opposite effect. Weak poses are body positions that make you smaller and more compact—for example, when you hunch over your notes to make a few last minute changes or when you cross your legs or arms.

Think about how you sit or stand before meeting with someone important or right before giving a talk. Do you stand tall (power pose) or sit with rounded shoulders (weak pose) as you read through your e-mail on your smartphone? If you must sit, turn your seated position into a power posture—that is, sit upright and keep your arms uncrossed by placing them on the arms of your chair. In the study, subjects who stood in weaker poses for a brief period of time had a 10% drop in testosterone and a 17% increase in cortisol levels. They felt less self-assured and decisive. Whatever you do, extend your limbs as much as possible for the greatest effect. If you can't physically strike one of these poses, picture yourself in one. Visualization is an effective tool you can use to help achieve success (Vasquez, 2007).

Respect Co-workers' Needs

We all interact with others in different ways. Some of us are introverted, whereas others are extroverted. Where do you and your co-workers lie on the introvert–extrovert continuum and how can you use this knowledge to communicate more effectively with one another?

- **If you are introverted:** You are energized by working alone. You prefer to speak up and share your thoughts after you first take time to prepare what you want to say. You enjoy devoting yourself to a single topic or activity, and you would rather socialize one-on-one than in a large group.
- **If you are extroverted:** You are energized when you work in groups, are assertive, are a go-getter, think well on your feet, and handle conflict well. You become energized in the company of others.

Whether you are a manager or staff member, respect your introvert-extrovert needs as well as those of your colleagues. If you are more extroverted, you may misinterpret an introverted colleague's quiet response as a sign that she is not interested in what you are saying. If you are introverted and invite a co-worker to coffee, you might feel inhibited or even slighted when he invites other co-workers to join you. Before you meet, make it clear that your get-together is just for the two of you.

All of us fall somewhere on the introvert-extrovert continuum depending on the topic, situation, and people around us. Sometimes we enjoy quiet and sometimes we love being in groups. But we tend to work best under certain conditions (Cain, 2012). It helps to understand your nature, so you can plan your interactions accordingly.

Know Your Thinking Style

We cannot safely assume that other people's minds work on the same principles as our own. All too often, others with whom we come in contact do not reason as we reason, or do not value the things we value, or are not interested in what interests us.

—Isabel Briggs Myers (1980)

According to the creators of the Myers-Briggs Type Indicator® (Briggs Myers, 1980), people come to conclusions by employing a combination of the following types of approaches: sensing, thinking, feeling, and intuition.

Sensing

Individuals who use sensing to help them arrive at decisions care more about the present than the future. They employ common sense to find solutions. They have a great memory for past events and facts, and they don't like to evaluate things if the details aren't clear.

Thinking

People who use thinking to help them assess a situation, turn to logic and proven data to make their decisions. They have a keen eye for what needs to be done. They believe that conflict between people is part of life.

Feeling

Those who employ feeling when they evaluate issues, consider not only how they feel about things, but also how other lives may be affected by their conclusions. They favor decisions that will be popular with others. Feeling individuals are uncomfortable with conflict.

Intuition

Individuals who use intuition to help them make decisions like to focus on the future. They have an active imagination and always consider new options. Once they understand a concept, they start to think of innovative ways to use it. They don't care if the presenting data aren't entirely clear, because they like to guess what the facts really show.

How do you make judgments? Which one of these combinations represents the way you perceive information: sensing plus thinking; sensing plus feeling; intuition plus thinking; or intuition plus feeling?

If you are a "sensing plus thinking" type of person and work with another "sensing plus thinking" employee, you likely will be on the same side of most, if not all, decisions. Every time an issue, such as budget allocation, comes up for debate, the two of you probably will be on opposite sides of the "intuitive plus feeling" co-workers. When you understand that those who don't agree with you merely have a different way of perceiving issues, you, hopefully, will be more understanding and less stressed by any conflicts that do arise and be more open to the thoughts and opinions of others.

Know Your History (Transference)

We discussed the value of knowing your history (transference) in Chapter 4. This information also can help you in the workplace. Have you ever had a co-worker who didn't like you regardless of how hard you tried to get along? Their resistance certainly could be from some recent perceived offense they have not yet shared, but also could reflect a relationship from their past. In most places of business, the boss is the head of the "work family." You and your co-workers are the "siblings" who compete for the boss' attention. The way your co-workers relate to one another often reflects how they interacted with their own siblings while growing up. For example, if Kirk is proud of you when your work is singled out by Dr. G, he probably reacted the same positive way when his own siblings received attention from their parents. If Loretta becomes jealous and then attempts to get her work praised also, it is very likely she responded with the same jealous behavior when one of her siblings took center stage. Everyone carries their history wherever they go. How did your family function?

If you become upset or feel jealous when a co-worker steals the limelight, consider your history as well as your coworker's history and engage in positive self-talk. Remember that sometimes, employees who are singled out as the boss' favorite don't want that position. If someone seems hostile after your boss praises you, stop, drop, and roll (SDR) and think compassionately about that person's need to be noticed and heard.

Consider Your Language

Now that you know more about your relationship and judgment style, have opened a window to your history, have agreed to be more honest with your coworkers, and are sitting or standing tall, you can begin to interact. When you speak, Adam Grant, PhD, a leading expert on success, motivation and giving, suggests you avoid the following "tentative markers" that can undermine your message (Grant, 2013):

Hedges

Hedges are words or phrases that people use to soften their messages. They don't add value to the statement itself, but can communicate uncertainty or ambivalence. "I was just wondering if you could" or "I sort of think you are right."

Hesitations

If you fill conversation pauses with words such as "well," "you know," "uh," and "um," you communicate anxiety and uncertainty. Some may respond sympathetically to your struggle to get your message out, but others may not. To help overcome this habit, relax before you speak. When you start to talk, slow your speaking pace and breathe. Tape yourself and listen to how you speak. Sometimes just becoming aware of the habit can help you do it less often.

Tag Questions

Tag questions are brief inquiry messages that many people tack on to the end of declarative statements: "That's interesting, *isn't it*?" "That's a good idea, *right*?" Tag questions soften what is being stated and invite others to agree or add their thoughts to the message. Tags also may hint that the speaker may lack confidence or doubt what they just said. To some, these questions can sound manipulative and devalue the speaker's message, although others may appreciate being asked their opinion.

Disclaimers

People use disclaimers to introduce their ideas: "this may not be the greatest idea, but" or "I'm not sure if this is really what you are looking for, but." Disclaimers can communicate uncertainty and might not keep people interested in what you have to say.

Verbosity Versus Directness

If you use more words than necessary to make a point, you make it harder for others to follow what you say. The more verbose you are, the greater the distance you put between yourself and your conversation partner. In this book, we often suggest that you ask your patients to respond to a question with one sentence or two. This helps them communicate more clearly and definitely saves time. Make an effort to be succinct also; your patients and co-workers will have an easier time hearing what you have to say. If you think that women are more verbose than men, you might be mistaken. According to a study conducted at the University of Arizona's Department of Psychology (Mehl, 2007), data analyzed from the voice recorders of 365 individuals showed that men and women both spoke approximately 16,000 words per day (our husbands vehemently disagree!).

Nonverbal Communication

The most important thing in communication is hearing what isn't said.
—Peter F. Drucker

People always communicate. As a matter of fact, you cannot *not* communicate. All of us share some of our thoughts through facial expressions, the clothes we wear, how we walk down the street, how we arrange our office space or home, our use of touch, vocal tone, and so on. Other types of nonverbal communication include hand gestures; posture; proximity to others; rate of speech; and whether we look, stare, or blink (Cherry, n.d.).

Some nonverbal behaviors seem easy to interpret, but they still can be misunderstood. Smiling, for example, can demonstrate happiness or pleasure, although the reason may not be obvious. Those who repeatedly glance at their watches may feel impatient or bored, or they may have somewhere they have to be that has nothing to do with you. Anxious or guarded individuals often cross their legs and arms, but so do many people who feel cold. When people turn their body away from another person, they often show ambivalence or simply are turning their attention to someone or something they find more interesting.

Most nonverbal messages are not clear, regardless of what popular books and magazines say. When you try to understand an action, consider the context of the conversation and the cultural background of the individual. The way various racial and ethnic groups use their eye contact and tone of voice differ. For example, African Americans, Asian Americans, and Latinos have nonverbal behaviors that are not shared by other groups (Lum, 2004). We glean as much as 80% of our understanding of messages from our *interpretation* of the nonverbal clues that accompany them (Roberson, 2010). So, if an action doesn't have a clear meaning or conflicts with what a person says, ask and clarify rather than assume that you know what the gesture means. That is the best way to limit misunderstandings and hurt feelings.

Because nonverbal messages can be misconstrued, be as clear both nonverbally and verbally as possible. When in doubt, ask the listener to tell you what they understood. This way you can see whether your message was received accurately and you will have an opportunity to correct any miscommunication. To ensure that your message is delivered properly, follow up with an e-mail that summarizes what you meant to convey. When your words are down in print, the recipient can review the information carefully and let you know if something is unclear.

"Fighting" Fair

Even if you fully appreciate your co-worker's differences, conflicts still can occur. As we said before, how you respond to others affects how others respond to you. Here are some guidelines that can help you and your co-worker deal with a conflict in a healthier way:

- Identify the problem
- Invite your co-worker to help set a time to discuss the problem. Ask, "Is now a good time to talk about this or after your next patient?" Let a bit of time pass between the argument and the discussion; it can help cool things down.
- When you meet, open by stating a positive goal: "I'd like us to find a way to work together, so we can be even more effective."
- Respect how you both feel about the issue. If you feel strongly, assume that your colleague feels strongly also. If you perceive things differently (i.e., sensing/thinking vs. intuition/feeling), you are less likely to see eye-to-eye on most things, at first.
- Even up the sides. If your colleague intimidates you, visualize yourself in a position of power. Imagine yourself standing on a chair carrying a loaded water pistol. Don't forget to strike a power pose for a minute or two before you meet.
- Attack the problem, *not* the person. Don't engage in derogatory name-calling. If you are tempted to do so, SDR!

- Breathe. The calmer you are, the better able you will be to deliver a clear message: SDR!
- Listen: don't interrupt each other.
- Use "I" statements, not blaming "You" statements. Do say: "I feel that" or "I need." Talk about *your* thoughts and actions, not what you expect your co-worker to think or do.
- If you don't resolve the problem, agree to disagree. The goal is not to lose or win, but rather to build a more effective way to interact and to understand each other's point of view.

How to Move On

After a tense interaction with a co-worker, you are likely to feel wound up. Breathe. Things may race through your head that you wished you had said, but didn't or couldn't. Breathe. Participate in positive self-talk: "I spoke honestly. I liked the way I stood my ground. I thought I did _____ really well. I could have done ____ better, but what I did made sense at the time." Keep a journal to clarify your feelings. Writing things down helps you vent and consider all that happened from a different perspective. Remember that it may take more than one conversation to resolve the problem.

Exercise also helps. John Ratey, a Harvard Medical School psychiatrist and author of *Spark: The Revolutionary New Science of Exercise and the Brain* (2008), states that "Exercise is the single best thing you can do for your brain in terms of mood, memory, and learning." It doesn't take a marathon to help you feel better. According to Ratey, as little as 10 minutes of exercise can alter your brain in a very positive way (Ratey, 2008).

When you head home, tell your loved ones about your day. Remind them that they don't have to provide you with answers, fix anything, or dislike the same person you do. You just need them to listen and be there for you. If you have a mentor, share your story with him or her. If not, consider getting one. Mentors can help you put things into perspective by sharing lessons learned from their own experiences. You can participate in peer supervision groups, if available, or create one of your own. If you feel the need, meet with a therapist who can help you identify your behavioral patterns as well as strengths. Therapists also offer a safe place to vent your anger and frustration, help you grow, and learn additional interaction skills.

Five-Minute Favors

Adam Rifkin, a successful entrepreneur, discovered a great way to build workplace relationships. He calls them "Five-Minute Favors." These are small acts of kindness that help you become "more bonded and attached to the people you're interacting with" (Huffington Post, 2013). The idea came to him after he observed several powerful, wealthy, and successful people doing small acts of kindness for others without expecting any benefit for themselves. When you take 5 minutes during the workday to do something nice for someone else, you get a great deal in return. We all have 5 minutes to spare in our workday. One thing you can do in 5 minutes is to introduce two colleagues. That takes very little time and can have a great impact in a friend's career. Another is to copy an article for a colleague or bring him or her a cup of coffee when you go for a fresh one of your own.

Bring Out the Best in Your Team

If you supervise employees, chair a committee, or are just part of a team, Appreciative Inquiry can help you motivate everyone to bring their best selves to the workplace. Like other strength-based techniques we have shared thus far, this problem-solving approach invites everyone to focus on what went well (WWW) and not on what needs to be fixed. Appreciative Inquiry "deliberately seeks to discover people's exceptionality—their unique gifts, strengths, and qualities. It actively searches and recognizes people for their specialties—their essential contributions and achievements . . . Appreciative Inquiry builds momentum and success because it believes in people" (Cooperrider, 2001).

Imagine you are seated in a hospital conference room. The head of your department enters and asks everyone to share problems that require attention. Immediately, everyone starts listing all that has gone wrong over the past few months: the rudeness of certain employees, the copier that constantly breaks down, and the co-worker who loses more messages than he passes on. By the end of the meeting, your team has identified a wealth of issues that require attention. Before you know it, you start to wonder why you still work here—the place is *so* awful. You feel disheartened and yearn to crawl back into bed.

Now, place yourself in the conference room once again. The department head enters, but makes a very different request. She first asks for any positive feedback members of your group have to share about the staff, the running of the department, or issues related to patient care. It could be their own thoughts or those of patients they have seen. Your colleague, Dr. Smith brings up Mrs. Johnson's comment (his patient) about how helpful everyone was when she came to the office on the wrong day. Next, the department head asks everyone to develop a list of things that are going *right*. What first comes to mind is the parking attendant who greets everyone with a warm, welcoming smile each morning. Next, you think of Dana, the receptionist who always puts patients at ease when they arrive. Again, the list grows, but it is filled with positive actions. When everyone is done, the chair gives you the second part of your assignment—to find ways to encourage these behaviors so they happen more often. As everyone brainstorms, you feel proud to be a part of an organization that values its employees and is doing so well.

Don't worry, even though they are not mentioned specifically, negative or difficult issues can be addressed with this approach. As Dana trains the office staff to be more helpful and supportive, those who answer the phones are more likely to deliver the messages they take. The staff member who is great at scheduling meetings, can schedule regular maintenance visits for the copier. "By studying the problems, we learn what 'not to do'" (Cooperrider, 2001). When we identify successes, we can build on what we know works well. Even if you are not in a position of power and your chairperson does not ask WWW, you can still raise your hand and contribute positive information to the discussion or ask to include it in future meetings.

The Takeaway

Encourage everyone to do more of what they do well, and make time to do "five-minute favors" for others. In the end, everyone wins!

9
All in the Family

I sustain myself with the love of family.
—Maya Angelou

In this chapter, you will learn the following:

- How to interact more effectively with your patients' families
- How to communicate more effectively with younger patients

After counseling an older gentleman about his diabetes, Janis escorted him to the lab where he took a seat. As she headed back to her office, she spotted a woman in the waiting area who was weeping silently. Janis introduced herself and asked if she could offer her any assistance. The woman identified herself as the wife of the man Janis had just seen. Then the woman leaned in and whispered the following call for help: "I can't take it anymore!" That emotion-filled moment and others Wendy also has observed in her practice prompted them to focus their practices and writings on ways to provide support to individuals with diabetes and their loved ones (Rapaport, 1989).

Working With Families

Diabetes doesn't exist in a vacuum. Picture a mobile dangling from a ceiling. Each piece represents your patient and members of his or her family. Now tap your patient's piece and consider what happens next—all the pieces begin to move. Some may swing more than others, but none stay entirely still. When one family member is diagnosed with diabetes, all are affected whether they wish to be or not. And what they do, what they say, and how supportive or unsupportive they are, affects your patients' ability to live with diabetes. How your patient responds to their help or lack of assistance affects other family members as well.

If certain relatives refuse to participate or show any interest in their loved one's diabetes that tells you something about the type of support your patients may or may not have. Use that information to direct your patients to alternative means of support, such as groups, one-on-one mentoring, and online support. If your patients don't want their family to come, respect their feelings, but help them explore their resistance. If needed, the therapist on your team should be able to assess if bringing their family in is a worthwhile goal.

Before You Meet

Before you schedule any family sessions, examine how your patients perceive the level of support they currently receive from their loved ones. Do they think it is reliable or absent? If a patient's family is supportive, he or she is fortunate as individuals with "warm, accepting and close" families adhere to medical recommendations three times more than those with less supportive families (DiMatteo, 2004). Supported patients are more likely to have better glycemic control (Pereira, 2008). In one longitudinal study, individuals with diabetes experienced an average drop of 4.9% in their A1C levels from preintervention to 1 month postintervention after their family members joined them in a diabetes education program. The subjects also enjoyed significant improvements in their "systolic blood pressure, diabetes self-efficacy, diabetes knowledge, and physical and mental components of health-related quality of life" (Hu, 2013). In addition, they consumed healthier foods and performed more blood glucose checks and foot inspections. If your patients hesitate to invite their family members to join them at an appointment, share this information.

Less supportive family members or loved ones can cause patients to feel alone or nagged and criticized. Conflicts are likely to arise when these patients try to introduce healthier behaviors into their home—for example, if they wish to eat healthier, but their relatives don't want to follow their lead (Gallant, 2007). Regardless of the level of support, encourage your patients to discuss their family issues with the health psychology member of their diabetes team, with a trusted member of the clergy, or with you at an additional appointment. This person can help them learn how to communicate their diabetes concerns more effectively. The therapist also may invite your patients to bring their families to one or more sessions to learn how they can support one another.

Now that you have an inkling of what to look for when you meet your patient's clan, set up the appointment. Let the family know the number of people you can accommodate at one time. Once a patient brought so many of her family members to meet with Janis that the small exam room began to feel like a circus clown car. So much time was spent shoving elbows and moving everyone around that very little appeared to be accomplished. But something wonderful did come of that session—the patient felt very supported and loved because so many of her family members showed up.

Use the stop, drop, and roll (SDR) intervention to take care of any negative feelings you may have toward any of your patients' relatives. Remind yourself that the negative stories your patients may have shared about their relatives are subjective and may not represent the real situation. Be sure to SDR if you feel angry because you've heard that some of the relatives contradict your advice. Again, these comments may not be accurate.

Time to Meet

Once you have calmed your own feelings, head into the room, and employ the LEAP approach to listening, which we discussed earlier:

- Listen to what the family members have to say.
- Empathize with them. Appreciate how frustrating it must be to love someone who has diabetes and doesn't take care of it as well as you or they feel they should.
- Affirm that their feelings and behaviors are common. Many relatives feel this way.
- Positively reframe their "meddling and criticizing" as evidence that they care and love their relative with diabetes.

Use your body language (eye contact, face the speaker, etc.) to demonstrate interest. If you are comfortable, use humor to get everyone's attention—ring a bell or hold up a stop sign. Don't be discouraged if the family is chaotic and struggles to settle down. Their behavior provides you with important information about how they interact. To help quiet the session, search for the leader in the room (a father, grandfather, mother, etc.) and enlist that person's help. Assure your patients' relatives that you are giving their loved one the most up-to-date medical information available and that you have asked them to contact you and other members of the diabetes team when questions arise.

When Waters Get Rough

Families may blame you for the difficulties they've experienced because of others in the medical system. They may accuse you of mismanaging their loved ones and argue that had you cared for them properly in the first place, they wouldn't have developed any complications. When this happens, SDR, so you can feel compassion, not anger or frustration. If your patients or family members claim to know more than you do, don't take their comments as personal attacks. Don't be defensive. SDR, SDR, SDR! Then say, "I respect all the work that you have done to find that information. I'm impressed that you know this." Even if there is a part of you that feels guilty, this conversation is not about you, it is about them and their feelings. So, positively reframe their arguing as a sign of how enthusiastically they care. And LEAP. When you listen to your patients' complaints without judgment, you give them an opportunity to feel some relief. Think of your efforts as healing, because they truly are.

As the family session continues, things may get heated and you will need to redirect everyone back to the purpose of the session—that is, to help their loved one. If you must quiet the room, SDR (to prepare yourself) and then say one or more of the following: "You all came today—that's love." "I'm happy to observe what your family is like." "I think you are hearing a lot of criticism and anger, but I'm also hearing a lot of love." If they remain silent and unresponsive, positively reframe their quiet response as a sign that they are thinking deeply about everything that is happening in the session.

Relatives

Relatives of people with diabetes have their own set of concerns and behaviors. You can help ease many of them when you provide accurate diabetes information and follow the LEAP approach when you speak with them. Many siblings worry that they will develop diabetes. Younger children often believe they caused their brother or sister's diabetes in some way (Rolland, 1994). Others may become jealous when their sibling with diabetes receives special attention.

They often feel guilty because they resent someone who has real medical needs. They also can feel overwhelmed if their parents ask them to "police" some of the behaviors of their sibling with diabetes.

Aunts and uncles as well as close friends (who are often like family) may urge your patients to skip painful or difficult self-care tasks, because they feel sorry about all they must do each day to care for their diabetes. Grandparents may feel inadequate and not invite their grandchild with diabetes to visit or spend the night; they fear they can't handle any emergencies that arise. Blended and single-parent families have their own unique issues, and parents who feel a range of emotions, including guilt, anger, and frustration, may berate you for not doing all they think you should do. If they insult or offend you, SDR and listen to them with additional compassion.

As professionals, we set the tone. From the very start, let your patients and supportive loved ones know that they are entitled to their feelings (even the negative ones). Life with diabetes is challenging, so it is as important to share, empathize, and affirm the entire spectrum of feelings everyone has without judgment, critique, or self-blame. Adolescents, unintentionally or intentionally, express their frustration in ways that can anger, frustrate, and upset their parents. Encourage everyone to SDR and LEAP, just as you do.

Explore Cultures

As your discussion continues, explore the family's cultural understanding of diabetes. In Chapter 3, we suggested you ask your patients the following questions. Ask their families the same questions (Anderson, 2002):

- What does having diabetes mean to you?
- What does having diabetes mean in your family?
- What does having diabetes mean in your community?

Their responses will help you connect to their value system. It is much easier to collaborate when you show respect for their values rather than trying to change them:

Gale and her family believe that a Higher Power controls healing. Initially, Craig, her endocrinologist, was frustrated by their lack of support for the self-care behaviors he and his diabetes team encouraged Gale to do each day—daily foot inspections, blood glucose checks, and insulin/carb ratios to estimate how much insulin to take throughout the day. Then, after using

SDR to control his growing anger, Craig enlisted their support by suggesting that diabetes self-care is a tool the Higher Power in the universe offers to help people heal. He also added that "man has been given wisdom to provide treatment. We are grateful for these options that can improve the quality of our life and help us to continue to serve and contribute to each other" (Anderson, 2002). His connecting to the family's value system made a difference. They all felt heard and respected and began to support many of the team's suggestions.

Be open to hearing about the cultural healing practices your patient's family endorses, such as Qigong, a walking form of Chinese meditation. Some studies demonstrate its role in improving diabetes control (Freire, 2013). Your open attitude models how one can have treatment preferences, yet still accept other options. If you find their beliefs too challenging to accept or believe that a certain practice may harm your patient or derail all that you want to do, SDR. Then share your concerns. Remember that their desire to have their loved one treat his or her diabetes using only traditional means comes from a place of love and caring. When you connect to that, it, hopefully, will be easier to communicate reliable information.

Marriage and Intimate Partnerships

As health care professionals, we often rely on spouses and intimate partners to support our patients' efforts to eat healthy, lose weight, take medications, and meet exercise goals. We also look to these devoted individuals to care for their loved ones emotionally when life with diabetes gets particularly tough. Being intimately involved with someone who has a chronic disease can be highly rewarding, but it also may be stressful at times.

Sometimes, partners can be so worried about their loved ones with diabetes that they begin to micromanage every health-related act they do. This heightened concern, which usually originates from a very loving place, can transform them into diabetes police officers and shift their loving partnerships into parent–child relationships. To help the couple rebalance their partnership and reduce the need for the diabetes police to appear, invite them to communicate more openly about their wants and needs by using the Daily Temperature Reading, an effective couple's communication tool we discuss in detail in Chapter 10. For additional ways to handle the diabetes police, we recommend materials available from http://www.behavioraldiabetes.org and Dr. William H. Polonsky's classic book, *Diabetes Burnout: What to Do When You Can't Take It Anymore* (1999).

Intimacy Issues

No matter how well couples communicate with one another, the diabetes in their lives is not going to disappear and may find its way into their bedroom.

About 50% of your male patients will experience physical, emotional, or hormonal issues, such as impeded blood flow, neuropathy, a low testosterone level, reduced self-esteem, and reduced libido that negatively affect their ability to achieve a satisfactory erection and enjoy intimacy (Roszler, 2007; Verschuren, 2010). Approximately 38% of your sexually active female patients likely will have decreased vaginal lubrication, reduced libido, self-esteem issues, require more time to become aroused, or a slight increased risk of dyspareunia (painful intercourse), even with good glucose control (Enzlin, 2009; Giugliano, 2010; Roszler, 2007; Verschuren, 2010). They are also more likely to experience increased vaginal infections but should be able to decrease the incidence with improved glucose control (Roszler, 2007). Difficulties in the bedroom can cause tension to develop between a couple that can reverberate throughout other areas of their life together. Here is one example:

> Dave rejected his wife, Laura's, sexual advances because he was afraid he wouldn't get an adequate erection. Laura felt rejected and angry. When he continued to behave this way without any explanation, she started to worry that he was having an affair. At Dave's appointment, his dietitian asked Laura to carefully read product labels so she could fill their pantry with healthier food options. Laura smiled and agreed to do what Dave's dietitian asked, but had no intention of following through. She was still too angry.

If you aren't comfortable discussing intimate topics, remind yourself that you have the ability to truly make a difference in your patients' lives by opening up the topic to discussion and providing them with reliable information and referral contacts. You can also encourage your patients to read *Sex and Diabetes: For Him and For Her* (Roszler, 2007), an entertaining and informative book that was nominated for Consumer Book of the Year (2008) by the Society for Sex Therapy and Research. This ADA publication not only explains diabetes-related sexual issues in clear, easy-to-understand language, it offers a wealth of creative ways to bring fun back into the bedroom when diabetes and complications are present. It also offers diabetes-friendly recipes that use aphrodisiac ingredients.

When Janis meets with health care professionals, she offers the following way to overcome the awkwardness of what often feels like an "invasion" of your patients' privacy:

> Compile a list of possible diabetes-related complications with your patient. When you mention sexual complications, stop for a moment and wait. Give your patient an opportunity to react. Those who don't have problems in this area are likely to respond by saying, "Oh, that's not me, thank goodness!" Or something similar, while those with difficulties will often ask for additional information.

You also can open the discussion with the diabetes-related sexual complications assessment quizzes we included in the references and resources section of this book. If you continue to struggle with this task, try to understand where your hesitancy comes from and talk yourself through it. Remind yourself that many of your patients need you to open the conversation and provide them with help or resources that can help them maintain or reclaim a satisfying intimate life. The more you talk about these topics, the more comfortable you and your patients will feel.

Loss and End-of-Life Issues

At some point, some of your patients and relatives will ask you to respond to questions about diabetes-related complications and death. These issues can be extremely difficult to discuss. Professor Nathan Katz, founder and director of the innovative Program in the Study of Spirituality at Florida International University, teaches students at Florida International University's medical school how to engage in an end-of-life conversation. According to Katz, "One cannot deal effectively with dying patients until one has made peace with one's own mortality. It is a challenge to get young medical students to look inward, but precisely that is the task at hand" (Nathan Katz, e-mail message to author, 2 December 2013). Certainly all of the listening steps we have shared with you throughout this book will help you connect with your patients and their families if and when this type of conversation takes place, but you must consider your own feelings about the issue. What do you believe about death? You don't have to share your personal opinions, but if you feel unsure, confused, or upset about the topic, it will make it harder for you to focus on your patients and their families. As with the sexual issues mentioned earlier, the more comfortable you are with this issue, the better you will be able to comfort those in need. Again, the more you understand your attitudes toward these issues, the better you will be able to assist your patients.

Patients may become angry because they want you to have all the answers when it comes to questions about suffering and loss. Their need for answers gives you an opportunity to remind them that they can reach out to various spiritual and religious institutions for guidance as well as to the health psychology professional on their diabetes care team. If you feel attacked by your patients or any of their relatives, SDR. They are stressed and want a place to release their fear and anger. You happen to be the authority figure who is either at the right place at the right time or was targeted as the recipient of their rage. Unfortunately, patients with problems that cannot be resolved medically often feel abandoned by their health care providers (Parker-Pope, 2010). Appreciate their need to have you listen to their concerns. You do that when you LEAP. Also, seek the assistance of the therapist on your team for the family and for yourself when these matters arise.

Kids' Behaviors

Following are some guidelines to help you interact more effectively with younger patients (De Jong, 2008):

Ask Strength-Based Questions

Many people respond negatively to questions that focus on what they are doing wrong, such as those that begin with the word "Why?" This is because the word "why" challenges; it is confrontational. Children tend to be especially sensitive to it. When worded positively, your question helps show respect and interest. Replace *"Why* didn't you check your blood this morning?" or *"Why* did you skip lunch yesterday?" which focus on what the child did wrong, with "How come?" *"How come* you missed lunch today?" The words "how come" show interest, but are softer and don't resonate as intensely. When you do this, use your body language to show sincere interest (eye contact, turn your body towards your patient, etc.) and don't judge or appear angry. Always assume that your young patients have a good reason (in their own minds) for doing a particular behavior. Remember when we discussed the young man who didn't check his blood because he didn't want to upset his mother? That was one reason that he had not been testing his blood glucose. Another reason could be that this teenager hates feeling bad when his results are not in a healthy range or that he doesn't want to appear different from his friends. Your job is to listen without judging and then help your patients learn a better way to understand the situation (remember Carl Rogers!).

How to Respond to "I Don't Know!"

Children, especially adolescents, who don't want to converse with an educator or health care provider, often will respond to questions by shrugging their shoulders and saying, "I don't know." If you follow up by asking more questions, you are likely to hear, "I don't know" again and again. When faced with this, keep calm. Remind yourself to SDR, so you can maintain a positive attitude toward them. Don't assume that these young patients are purposely trying to be difficult. They actually may not know the answer to your question or may be afraid to respond in front of their parents. So set aside some time to speak with them privately. But start the session with the parents present, so you can gain their trust. They also can provide you with information that will help you guide their child. When you meet with them, encourage them to focus on their child's goals and accomplishments (Affirmative Inquiry) and direct them away from seeing negative actions as misbehavior.

If a child hesitates to answer you, gently and sincerely respond by saying, "I realize that I'm asking some tough questions. [Pause.] So, suppose you did know, what would you say?" This unexpected response usually will prompt them to say something—remind them that there are no right or wrong answers. Another option is to invite them to consider another viewpoint. Ask, "What would your best friend say?" When you mention their best friend, you bring a very important person into the conversation—a best friend has their back. He or she supports them and accepts them as they are. When you invite them to share what their best friend may think, they may provide you with insightful information. If you think it would be helpful, you can suggest that their best friend attend the next session to offer additional emotional support (Palladino, 2012).

If nothing works and "I don't know" or total silence is the only response your young patients are willing to give, don't get frustrated. SDR. Try to consider the interaction from a compassionate and positive perspective. They may not answer you because they have been taught to think carefully and don't want to respond to a question before they are certain of the answer. Their reluctance to respond may indicate that they have a strong will and are determined, both of which can help them live well with their diabetes; it takes a lot of effort to stay quiet when adults urge you to say something. Don't be afraid to join them in their silence. It may feel awkward at first, but when a child chooses to be silent and you sit there, quietly, as if you have nothing else to do, you communicate an acceptance of the child's choice to stay quiet. Let them know that you appreciate that they must have good reasons not to talk; you respect their decision to respond this way. Some children need to have this acceptance before they feel comfortable enough to open up. If keeping silent is tough for you, share the positive thoughts you have about their silence: "I like that you are taking your time and only want to answer when you are ready." Sometimes children need time to examine their motivations. You can help them explore.

Adolescents

Think back to what life was like when you were an adolescent— peer pressure, bullying (now cyberbullying), puberty, romantic crushes, broken hearts, driving, and, of course, a strong desire to be independent—not to mention risky behaviors, lying, and certain rites of passage in some teens (drinking, irresponsible driving, stealing, sexual acting out, preoccupation with body image, etc.). Throw in a whirlwind of social and emotional changes plus diabetes and communication can be a real challenge. If you work with adolescents, retain close contact with their parents throughout and encourage them to support their teen every step of the way. Initially, we believed that teens needed to separate from their parents as they grew and became independent custodians of their diabetes (Anderson, 2000). But that perspective has changed. We now understand that parents should "foster autonomy while staying involved" (Anderson, 2012).

Encourage parents (and remind yourself) to react positively when a teen comes in with negative glucose test results. Say, "It is great that you tested. These results can help you learn a lot about your diabetes. The 300 g/dl result you got yesterday afternoon explains at least part of why you feel so tired a lot of the time. (*Empathy.*) Let's talk about decisions you can make to help you feel more energized throughout the day."

Parents and even siblings likely will feel increased levels of stress when a family member is diagnosed with diabetes. Some parents may find it helpful to attend group or private parenting classes to learn how to communicate health concerns without criticizing, how to deal with feelings of guilt or sadness, how to communicate with school staff, and more. The diagnosis of diabetes can provide an opportunity for other family issues to be explored, such as marital disharmony or an overly critical and chaotic home environment. Some parents unconsciously focus on their children's medical issues as a way to deflect attention from less healthy family behaviors. If this seems to be the case, bring in a health psychology professional to help you introduce the family to additional and more intensive counseling.

Following are some communication strategies that can help you and your adolescent patient interact more effectively:

- **Speak respectfully.** It is tempting to speak to a 12-year-old in the same way you might speak to a 7- or 8-year-old, but adolescents respond more enthusiastically when you speak to them as if they were adults. They may not be able to think as maturely as adults do, but they want to be treated in an adult way.

- **Keep your words to a minimum.** If you are a fan of Peanuts cartoons, you might recall how Charlie Brown and his gang were portrayed when their antics were televised. When their teacher spoke in the classroom scenes, all the kids heard was "Wah-wah-wah-wah." They tuned out and didn't hear much of what she said. If you lecture or go on too long with an explanation, your words are likely to have little, if any, impact (Faber, 2010). A better strategy is to ask your young patients to share what they know about a particular topic and comment on their words.

- **LEAP.** The same approach that we touted for your other patients works with teens as well. They want to be heard and the LEAP approach helps you communicate respect and shows that you value what your teen patient has to say. When you include the entire family, you have an opportunity to listen to everyone who plays a role in your adolescent patient's care and can develop goals together. According to Brian (n.d.), "Talking to a teen isn't just about talking. It's about listening. They are going through physically, mentally, emotionally and physiologically demanding changes. Teens may seem incredibly melodramatic, but they still need to be listened to."

- **What Went Well (WWW).** When you meet with the parents of your young patients, invite them to tell you what their child does well and what behaviors they would like to see their child do more often. If you recall from our discussion of Appreciative Inquiry (see Chapter 8), when you focus on what is going well, you also take care of problematic issues. Discuss their children's strengths while the children are present. It can be empowering for your patients to hear the positive things others say about them as it helps them experience new ways to perceive themselves and their issues (Freedman, 1996). Excuse the parents from the room and then spend time alone with the child or teen. At the end of the session, invite the parents to return and have their children summarize what they gained from meeting with you.

Find out what your young patients care about and develop goals together. Be open to why they may or may not want to do certain tasks. If you have difficulty believing the information they share, consider past relationships or experiences you've had that may cause you to be especially wary of the comments young patients say. Were your adolescent children honest with you? Perhaps you weren't very forthcoming with your own parents when you were that age. Identify any *transference* issues that you may bring with you to the session and SDR. Know your history (see Chapter 4). Then be open to the responses these young patients give. They deserve your attention and support. Your adolescent patients are trying to find their way in a challenging world with diabetes as their constant companion. When you have their trust, you can help guide them. Utilize the talents of the health psychology professional on your team to help the family adjust as more responsibility is given to their child. They may find support groups at your center or in your community helpful as well.

The Takeaway

Don't treat your patients in a vacuum. Include their family.

10
Heading Home

I n this chapter, you will learn the following:

- How to transition from work to home mode
- Effective ways to enhance your personal connections outside of the office

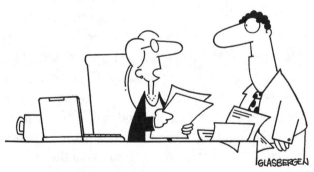

Copyright 2001 by Randy Glasbergen.
www.glasbergen.com

GLASBERGEN

"You could call me a workaholic if I brought my
work home with me, but I don't go home!"

It's late, a lot later than you (and your family) probably want it to be, but you finally are headed home. How can you let go of your role at work and the pressures that go along with it and segue into the next phase of your day? We suggest you start by doing the following:

Ritualize Quitting Time

Remember how each Flintstone's cartoon began? Fred was seated high atop a dinosaur, digging away in the quarry. Suddenly the quitting time bird would crow and off Fred would go, sliding down his dinosaur's back to head home. Unlike Fred, however, many of us never stop working. Even after we leave the office, we continue to behave as if we were still on the clock. We respond to e-mails, text colleagues, answer phone calls, and continue with office projects. We reflect on issues we handled and decisions we made. We might even worry about what we have planned for tomorrow. If you work without end, you are at risk for developing a whole list of stress-related issues. You can harm important family relationships if you allow your work to interfere with the quality time you set aside for your loved ones. Self- care is one of the top 10 things you can do to help prevent burnout (Linzer, 2014), so take care of your emotional health and disconnect from your workday by ending it at a specific time, in a specific way.

Sound the Whistle

Identify a moment when you officially "call it a day." It could be when you close your office door, exit your building, or start the engine of your car in the parking lot. If you work from home, it is even more critical to choose a specific stopping point as your workday can go on, uninterrupted, well into the night. Once you pick a closing time, ritualize it. Do some action that marks it as a real endpoint. One way to do this is to stop for a moment and breathe. Not only is breathing calming (as we mentioned in Chapter 1), but also it can shift you into a "much more peaceful frame of mind" (Borysenko, 2011). Breathe like a baby does: inhale and expand your belly, exhale and contract your belly. If you listen to music as you head home, you join a long tradition of using music to relieve stress that dates back to 4000 B.C. and may even go all the way back to Paleolithic times (Horden, 2000). If you are spiritual, say a personal prayer for all of the lives you touched that day and be grateful for the type of work you do. Ritualizing this moment helps you move to the next phase.

If you are running late, call ahead to let your loved ones at home know that you are on your way. If they respond with annoyance, listen to their comments and use the stop, drop, and roll (SDR) intervention. Consider what it must be like for them to wait for you. Don't react to their frustration. If necessary, let them know that you appreciate how hard this is for them—never take their support for granted. You have behavioral options, so *choose* to remain in a positive mood as you head home.

Transition: Review Your Day

As a healer, thinker, innovator, and communicator, your day can become hectic. Once you locate your endpoint and ritualize it, engage in positive self-talk to help tie up any emotional loose ends and calm any lingering nerves. Here's how:

- Make a mental or actual list of what went well (WWW) today. In a previous chapter, we discussed the concept of Affirmative Inquiry and how focusing on the positive resolves negative issues as well. You do a number of things well each day. Take time to remember those things. Choose not to dwell on things that went awry or what you could have done better. If you feel compelled to revisit the negative parts of your day, limit your mental review to 5 minutes. If a certain problem troubles you further, set a time to address it in more depth with your boss, a peer, or even with a therapist. Don't ruminate over it; remember that communication is circular—it is highly unlikely that the negative interaction was entirely your fault. Be mindful of the positive role you can play in future interactions.
- Recognize your impact. You affect many lives, even some you may not know about. One patient might share your advice with a friend or a family member. A visitor may have been so impressed by your professional demeanor that she made an appointment at your center. A colleague may have been inspired after seeing how well you interacted with a patient. You never know whose lives you have touched.
- Forgive yourself for being human. No one is perfect and you attempted to do your best. If you did something you regret, what can you learn from it and how can you use that insight to respond differently next time?
- If you owe someone an apology, first give yourself a pat on the back for accepting the fact that no one, including you is perfect. Then make a mental note to call or speak to that person at an appropriate time. Apologizing does not show weakness and it does not mean you were necessarily wrong. It shows that you are now more aware of the impact your behavior had on that particular interaction. It also shows

your strength and desire to change. There is no way to know whether the person you offended will accept your apology, but that shouldn't stop you from doing what you believe is right. If you encourage your patients and others to be true to themselves, you should do the same. Follow your own advice.

Be Mindful

If you still feel stressed when you arrive home, turn off your work-related electronics. Don't be surprised if you have difficulty doing this; many people do. According to Oulasvirta (2012), people who use mobile devices can develop a very repetitive and annoying "checking habit," which is defined as a "brief, repetitive inspection of dynamic content." You may be tempted to decompress and numb uncomfortable feelings by sitting at your home computer, watching some television, snacking, or drinking an alcoholic beverage. Instead, employ one of the tools you used to start your day—that is, mindfulness. It can help you reduce your stress and deal more effectively with troubling thoughts. Mindfulness, as we mentioned earlier, does the exact opposite of what television shows and computer games do—it invites you to pay attention to your thoughts, not to distract yourself from them. That may sound counterintuitive, but it is anything but. Increasing your awareness of issues that bother you can help you resolve them later. When you set aside time to pay closer attention to your body, your breathing, and the thoughts that pass through your mind, you can reduce your stress and increase your feeling of well-being (Brown KW, 2003). Studies show that improved mindfulness also can reduce anxiety, pain, hot flashes, and help individuals with a history of major depression avoid relapses (Harvard Mental Health Letter, 2011).

How mindful are you? If you often bump into things, spill drinks, and multitask while others speak to you, you are probably not very mindful. You could also benefit from mindfulness-strengthening exercises if you have a hard time focusing on things around you, end up at your work parking lot without knowing how you got there, rush through most tasks, or snack without even noticing that you are eating. To become more mindful, try the following mindfulness stress reduction exercise recommended by the authors of the Harvard Mental Health Letter (2011). Share this information with others or invite someone you care about to do it with you:

Step 1. Center Down

Sit down on the floor (cross-legged) or on a sturdy, straight-backed chair and breathe. Notice how the air enters your nose and exits your mouth. Feel your abdomen expand and contract as you breathe in and out.

Step 2. Open Up

While seated, pay attention to the sounds in your environment and the different sensations you feel. Don't worry if ideas start to pop into your mind. When they do, think about each for a moment and then let it go. If ideas start to overwhelm you, focus on your breathing once again.

Step 3. Observe

Observe what enters your mind. As you hear sounds and feel different sensations, let them pass. Notice how you respond to different thoughts. Become aware of the things that enhance your feeling of well-being and those that make you feel uncomfortable. Just observe it all.

Step 4. Stay with It

At times, you may not feel relaxed when you do this, but stick with it. Most of us are not used to being mindful. We are too busy with our hectic lives and with all of the technological demands on us: our cell phones, computers, and other personal devices. Take time each day to do this mindfulness exercise. If possible, build up to 20–45 minutes. The more you do it, the better you will feel.

Do As I Say, Not As I Do

As a health care professional, you probably have a long list of healthy activities you encourage patients to try to reduce their stress. *Take your own advice!* If you encourage your patients to be physically active, do that too. If you find it hard to fit exercise into your day, take that awareness with you to work and be more compassionate as you SDR after a patient shares that she didn't stick to your physical activity prescription. Gone are the days when health care advisors can be overweight smokers and demand that their patients lose weight and quit smoking. Be congruent: Do what you say and say what you do. Let your patients motivate you as you motivate them.

Behaviors at Home

At work, your patients and colleagues value you for your expertise. Patients look to you to help them solve problems in their lives and colleagues turn to you for advice. When you get home, you may not engender the same respect. The transition from your expert position at work to driving a carpool and taking out the garbage can be a tough one. Appreciate the impact you have outside of work. Focus on the emotional "high" you can get from being a loving partner, parent, and friend.

What happens when you arrive home after a hard day of work? If you live with others and walk in unannounced, are you greeted warmly by loved ones (and perhaps a loyal pet) or do you find everyone in the middle of phone conversations, computer chats, or other activities? If you live alone, do you feel a need to reach out to friends and loved ones?

Queen Elizabeth rarely walks into a room without having someone announce that she is about to enter. The announcement gives everyone time to stop what they are doing and turn their attention toward her. You deserve to come home to a warm, welcoming "castle" of your own, but that is less likely to happen if you surprise everyone with your entrance. Call ahead and give them notice. When you arrive at your door one thing you certainly can do with your loved one is hug. Dr. David Schnarch, author of *Intimacy & Desire* (2009), is a huge fan of hugging, and so are we. Hugging not only helps reduce anxiety but also raises the body's oxytocin and feelings of trust by lowering the activation of our brain's amygdala, which controls fear (Pillay, 2010).

Schnarch recommends we hug our loved one until we feel relaxed. When done as described below, his "hugging till relaxed" tool becomes a "mindfulness activity, a way of centering yourself, quieting your mind, and getting control of your emotions—while you're close to your partner." Unlike romantic hugging, which is done to connect to your partner, this particular hug helps you and your loved one nurture your own needs as you support one another. Encourage your partner to enjoy the benefits of Schnarch's "hugging till relaxed" also.

1. Stand on your own two feet.
2. Put your arms around your partner.
3. Focus on yourself.
4. Quiet yourself down. *Way* down.

(Schnarch, 2009)

Enhancing Connections

We live hectic lives. Too often, we don't get a chance to share much of what happens during our day with our loved ones. If you have a significant other in your life and you fail to connect on a regular basis, you eventually may grow apart. According to John Gottman, a pioneer in the field of marital counseling, the negative effects of marital dissolution are quite extensive. They include an "increased risk of psychopathology; increased rates of automobile accidents, including fatalities; increased incidence of physical illness, suicide, violence, and homicide; decreased longevity; significant immunosuppression; and increased mortality from diseases" (Gottman, 1999).

The Daily Temperature Reading (DTR) is a wonderful activity that can help you and a loved one connect each day. It also can be done with others in your life. Virginia Satir developed the concept of a DTR, which the nonprofit PAIRS Foundation (at http://www.PAIRS.com) adapted and features in the relationship skills classes it has taught to tens of thousands of people over the past 30 years. The DTR takes about 15–20 minutes. The PAIRS Foundation website also offers a DTR app, so you can complete the activity using your smartphone. DTR includes five simple steps that you and your loved one can run through each day, or as often as possible. Give it a try. Not only have we enjoyed using it, but also the PAIRS Foundation has impressive research that supports its use as well as the use of other tools it teaches at its different classes (Peluso, 2011). Each of the five steps will help you and your loved one connect more deeply. Take turns as you go through the following sequence:

1. Appreciations
2. New information
3. Puzzles
4. Concerns with recommendations
5. Wishes, hopes, and dreams
   (With permission from PAIRS Foundation, 2013)

Appreciations

The first step opens your interaction on a positive note. Take turns saying one thing you appreciate about each other. Be very specific. Instead of saying something general such as, "I appreciate how nice you are to me," say, "I appreciate the delicious dinner you prepared. You took the time to make spaghetti, my favorite dish." A specific compliment communicates so much more. It shows that you were mindful and really noticed the action your loved one did.

New Information

Next, take turns and briefly mention something new that happened during the day. Did anything happen at work? Perhaps you ran into an old friend, or just read that the elliptical machine you want to buy is going on sale. Most of us spend a great deal of time apart from our loved ones. We connect when we share new information each day.

Puzzles

Many couples get derailed when they *assume* something without finding out if their assumption is correct. Here is what happened to Nick and Patty:

> While hosting a couple of friends for dinner, Patty abruptly got up and left the room. Nick immediately thought, "Oh, I bet Patty got offended when our friends made those nasty comments about the candidate we supported. We better not invite them over anymore." If Nick doesn't ask Patty why she left, he might act on his assumption and stop having these friends over. He might also feel embarrassed that he has a wife with poor manners. Nick and Patty DTR each day. When they reached this step, Nick said the following: "Patty, I noticed that you got up suddenly when our friends were visiting. How come you left during the political discussion we were having? Imagine Nick's surprise when Patty responded, "Oh, I wasn't even listening. I ate something spicy earlier that day and suddenly started to feel ill. You know how sensitive my stomach is sometimes. That's why I left." With that information, Nick now understands the situation better. Nothing has to change except for Patty's food choices! Don't assume. When you get to this step, each take a turn to inquire about something you are wondering about or don't understand.

Concerns With Recommendations

This is the time when you and your loved one can mention something you find troubling, but you are going to do it in a new way. Too often, when people criticize, they don't offer any solutions. When that happens, the recipient of their critique can feel attacked. By offering a suggestion along with your concerned comment, you turn a potentially hurtful moment into a problem-solving one, which is far more productive. When you make your comment, first focus on *your* perspective then make your recommendation. For example:

Doug always leaves his shoes by the front door, which really bothers his partner Roger. So Roger says, "When I come home from work and see your shoes by the front door, I feel bad because the rest of the house look so nice and clean. How about if I buy a decorative basket to put by the door? You could put your shoes in there." Doug responds, "I didn't know my shoes bothered you. Don't buy the basket, I'll try to put them away when I get home." Had Roger said, "I can't stand seeing your shoes everywhere! Where do you think we live . . . in a pigsty?" Doug would not have responded positively and a painful fight could have started.

Wishes, Hopes, and Dreams

We began the DTR with a positive appreciation and end it on a positive note as well. It means a lot to include your loved one in your dreams for the future. Each take a moment to say something that you hope to do one day in the future. It can be realistic or totally crazy. You can hope to buy that house you've always wanted, learn to play the ukulele, or sail around the world. Include your loved one in your dream, if desired. When we share our hopes and dreams with our loved ones, we continue to picture them in our future. Visit http://www.PAIRS.com for more information about the DTR and other relationship enhancement tools and classes.

Support Your Efforts

Don't underestimate the value of a minivacation to support your efforts to calm down and recharge your emotional and physical batteries. Observant Jews, for example, take a minivacation each week when they observe the Sabbath. From sundown Friday evening, until sundown Saturday night, these Sabbath observers separate themselves from the rat race of the regular world. They don't talk on the phone, use computers, watch television, write, open mail, or do other business-related activities. Instead, they pray, study religious topics, go on walks, visit friends, play board games, and rest. You don't have to go to that extreme, but you still can benefit from taking a personal minivacation, such as a weekend getaway at a local hotel or ski lodge, or an electronic minivacation by turning off your smartphone, computer, tablet, and other tools for a period of time. You can also schedule non-work-related events into your week, such as a concert, lecture, or book club discussion. Be sure to take the official vacation you are given each year from your workplace as "skipping vacations can lead to a loss of productivity and creativity, negatively impact the quality of your work and eventually cause burnout" (Rubin, 2012).

Take Our Approaches Home

Throughout this book, we've shared options you can use with behaviors at your workplace. Don't leave them at the office. Use them at home and in other areas of your life, so all your interactions become more meaningful. Nancy, a diabetes educator, says she has incredible patience at work. "I can listen to my patients all day!" But when it comes to her husband, she is always upset about something. When he arrives home from work, the nasty comments and digs roll off her tongue. She hates being the shrew. She really wants to welcome him in a loving way, but she says she switches into some horrible default mode when he walks in the door. Living that way is exhausting. Home should be a place to unwind and feel safe, so you and your loved ones can recharge and reconnect. If you are unable to relax and be yourself at home, it makes it harder to bring your best self to work each day. Nancy owes it to herself and her husband to be as compassionate at home as she is at work.

Use the interactive approaches you've learned from this book at home as well. Apply the SDR intervention to calm yourself when your teen asks for money. SDR when you go to the cleaners and find that they lost your favorite dress. Listen, empathize, affirm, and positively reframe (LEAP) when a friend calls to complain about the escalating cost of the wedding she is planning for her daughter. Use affirmative language, such as "I" statements to communicate your thoughts, feelings, and needs. Employ other approaches (from Chapters 4 and 5) when different behaviors arise. The more you use these approaches, the more comfortable they will become and the more honest your relationships will be. Develop "emotional literacy"—that is, learn to recognize, empathize, understand, and competently handle and respond to your own emotions as well as to those of others around you (Goleman, 1997). When you convey how you really feel inside (your inside matches your outside), others always will know where you stand. Be authentic. Be genuine. Be congruent. What we do for ourselves, better enables us do for others.

Revisiting Peggy

In Chapter 1, we introduced you to Peggy. If you recall, she was a diabetes educator who had a particularly challenging day. Here is how her day was transformed after incorporating some of the approaches discussed throughout this book:

Peggy expected to have a tough morning, but surprised herself when she woke up before her alarm went off. The evening before, she and her husband enjoyed a light dinner then went for a brisk walk. While they were out, they ran through the daily temperature reading (DTR), which helped them share a few issues that were on their minds; they even straightened out a troubling money misunderstanding they had. During the wishes, hopes, and dreams step of the DTR, they chatted about their future plan to visit the Grand Canyon. That evening, after the great talk and quick walk, Peggy had no trouble falling asleep when bedtime rolled around.

The next morning, after hitting the snooze alarm repeatedly, Peggy dragged herself out of bed. The night before, she accepted the fact that she took a long time to wake up, so she reset her alarm to give herself a bit more time to lie lazily in bed (*slow down*). She smiled at how she could change her mood just by acknowledging and accepting her personal needs (*cognitive restructuring*). Then she tried on several outfits, each feeling too tight for the long day she had ahead. As expected, she started to berate herself for her current weight, but quickly told herself that today was a new day (*positive reframe/self-compassion/self-talk*). She even set out her sneakers and workout clothes, as a positive reminder that she planned to exercise later today. She texted her walking buddy as she prepared her breakfast, to remind her that they were definitely going to meet (*anticipate*). With her good health in mind, she looked past her husband's cookies and poured herself a bowl of whole grain cereal with berries. She was proud of herself for making a healthier choice (*self-talk/appreciation*).

Peggy and her husband shared a loving hug as they each went off to work (*gratitude*). Traffic was particularly heavy, so Peggy called ahead to let her co-workers know she was running late (*anticipate*). Now, she could relax as she sat in traffic and listen to her favorite drive-time radio show (*slow down*). When she arrived at the office, Dr. G was in a foul mood. The moment he saw Peggy, he ordered her to meet with Mrs. X, a patient who always got on his nerves, and then he rushed off to answer a call. Peggy took a moment to SDR. Usually, Dr. G was very considerate, so she assumed that something must be on his mind and she didn't take his harsh tone personally (*self-talk*). Before entering Mrs. X's exam room, Peggy stopped to SDR. She had heard that Mrs. X tested everyone's patience. She reminded herself that

Mrs. X struggled with her diabetes control and had little support at home. Her negative comments probably came from her frustration with both of those things. Next, Peggy entered Mrs. X's exam room and greeted her with a warm smile. Mrs. X responded to Peggy's positive mood. She smiled back and said, "I need to lose weight. Are you sure you can help me? You are just as overweight as I am!" (*Listen.*) Instead of being offended, Peggy laughed (*humor*). "You're right. I know how hard it is to lose weight (*empathy*). You're not alone (*affirm*). But I have had some success. I was actually quite a bit heavier, so let me tell you what's worked for me" (*self-disclosure/encouragement*). Mrs. X's face lit up. "Finally, someone who understands weight loss! Let's talk!" (*Humor*). What followed was a great conversation filled with laughter and great collaboration.

Later, Dr. G asked Peggy to share what happened with Mrs. X. Before entering his office, Peggy took a moment to SDR and reminded herself to be more compassionate about how Dr. G had treated her earlier. As she entered his office, smiling, he immediately responded with a smile and said, "Your session went well? I can't believe it!"

Peggy answered, "Mrs. X needed someone to listen to her first before she would be willing hear any information. I let her know that she isn't alone and that I have information that can help her (*affirm*). We had a terrific talk" (*WWW*).

"It sounds like you have the magic touch, Peggy," said Dr. G. "When we have a bit more time, I'd like to know exactly what you did to turn her around."

"Thank you" (*appreciation*). Peggy responded with a grin. "During our next break, I'll share what we did. If you are interested, I can also share some of the other new interaction approaches I learned" (*WWW*).

The Takeaway

Be authentic. Be genuine. Be congruent. Communicate openly, honestly, and empathically at work and in your personal life.

References and Resources

References

Adams P. Humour and love: the origination of clown therapy. *Postgrad Med J* 2002;78:447–448.

Al-Arouj M, Bouguerra R, Buse J, Hafez S, Hassanein M, Hassanein M, Ibrahim MA, Ismail-Beigi F, El-Kebbi I, Khatib O, Kishawi S, Al-Madani A, Mishal AA, Al-Maskari M, Ben Nakhi A, Al-Rubean K. Recommendations for management of diabetes during Ramadan. *Diabetes Care* 2009;28(9):2305–2311.

Allan R. *Getting Control of Your Anger; A Clinically Proven Three-Step Plan for Getting to the Root of the Problem and Resolving it.* New York, McGraw Hill, 2005.

American Association of Diabetes Educators. The AADE7™. Available at http://www.diabeteseducator.org/ProfessionalResources/AADE7. Accessed 3 June 2014.

American Diabetes Association. Association issues new nutrition therapy position statement. *Diabetes Pro* 2013 Fall;36(11):3821–3842.

American Diabetes Association. Nutrition recommendations and interventions for diabetes. *Diabetes Care* 2008;31(Suppl. 1):S61–S78.

American Psychological Association. Anger management, n.d. Available at http://www.apa.org/topics/anger/control.aspx#. Accessed 16 October 2013.

American Psychological Association. What you need to know about will-power. 2014. Available at https://www.apa.org/helpcenter/willpower.aspx. Accessed 26 May 2014.

Anderson B. Family teamwork and type 1 diabetes. Lecture, Friends for Life Conference; Orlando, Florida, 6 July 2012.

Anderson BJ, Harris MA. Working with adolescents and families. Paper presented at the 60th Scientific Sessions of the American Diabetes Association, San Antonio, Texas, 12 June 2000.

Anderson BJ, Rubin RR. *Practical Psychology for Diabetes Clinicians.* 2nd ed. Alexandria, VA, American Diabetes Association, 2002.

Anderson RT, Camacho FT, Balkrishnan R. Willing to wait? The influence of patient wait time on satisfaction with primary care. *BMC Health Serv Res* 2007;28(7):31–35.

Attia P. Who I Am. *The Eating Academy,* 2012. Available at http://eatingacademy. com/dr-peter-attia. Accessed 25 May 2014.

Baikie KA, Wilhelm K. Emotional and physical health benefits of expressive writing. *Adv Psychiatr Treat* 2005;11:338–346.

Baldwin K, Ginsberg P, Harkaway RC Under-reporting of erectile dys-function among men with unrelated urologic conditions. *Int J Impot Res* 2003;15(2):87–89.

Barnard K, Peveler RC, Holt RI. Antidepressant medication as a risk fac-tor for type 2 diabetes and impaired glucose regulation. *Diabetes Care* 2013;36(10):3337–3345.

Baumeister RF, Tierney J. *Willpower.* New York, NY, Penguin Group, 2011.

Bayne H, Neukrug E, Hays D, Britton B. A comprehensive model for opti-mizing empathy in person-centered care. *Patient Educ Counsel* 2013;93(2): 209–215.

Bègue L, Bushman BJ, Zerhouni O, Subra B, Ourabah M. Beauty is in the eye of the beer holder: people who think they are drunk also think they are attrac-tive. *Br J Psychol* 2012;104:225–230.

Bennett MP, Lengacher C. Humor and laughter may influence health: III. Laughter and health outcomes. *Evid Based Complement Alternat Med* 2008;5(1):37–40.

Berg CA, Butner JE, Butler JM King PS, Hughes AE, Wiebe DJ. Parental persuasive strategies in the face of daily problems in adolescent type 1 diabetes management. *Health Psychol* 2013;32(7):719–728.

Beukeboom CJ, Langeveld D, Tanja-Dijkstra K. Stress-reducing effects of real and artificial nature in a hospital waiting room. *J Altern Complement Med* 2012;18(4):329–333.

Borysenko J. Breathing, 2011. Available at http://www.youtube.com/watch?v=gVzuV2IBdNk. Accessed 2 December 2013.

Borysenko J. Save your breath and keep your sanity. *HuffPost Healthy Living,* 2008. Available at http://www.huffingtonpost.com/joan-borysenko/save-your-breath-and-keep_b_104971.html. Accessed 21 December 2013.

Boyes A. Cognitive restructuring. In practice, 2 January 2013. Available at http://www.psychologytoday.com/blog/in-practice/201301/cognitive-restructuring. Accessed 12 November 2013.

Bremner RH, Koole SL, Bushman BJ. "Pray for those who mistreat you": effects of prayer on anger and aggression. *Pers Soc Psychol Bull* 2011;37(6):830–837.

Brewer J. How to face fear. *Huffington Post Healthy Living,* 2013. Available at http://www.huffingtonpost.com/dr-judson-brewer/fear-and-motivation_b_3558490.html. Accessed 24 October 2013.

Brian P. How to talk to a teen. *Psychology Dictionary,* n.d. Available at http://psychologydictionary.org/article/how-to-talk-to-a-teen/. Accessed 8 December 2013.

Briggs Myers I, Myers PB. *Gifts Differing: Understanding Personality Type.* Mountain View, CA, CPP Inc., 1980.

Brown B. *The Gifts of Imperfection: Let Go of Who You Think You're Supposed to Be and Embrace Who You Are.* Center City, MN, Hazelden Publishing, 2010.

Brown KW, Ryan RM. The benefits of being present: mindfulness and its role in psychological well-being. *J Pers Soc Psychol* 2003;84(4):822–848.

Buchanan L. Leadership advice: strike a pose. *Inc Magazine.* May 2012 Available at http://www.inc.com/magazine/201205/leigh-buchanan/strike-a-pose.html. Accessed 22 September 2013.

Cain S. *Quiet: The Power of Introverts in a World that Can't Stop Talking.* New York, NY, Crown Publishers, 2012.

Cain S. The power of introverts, n.d. Available at http://www.ted.com/talks/susan_cain_the_power_of_introverts.html. Accessed 20 September 2013.

Carney DR, Cuddy AJ, Yap AJ. Power posing. Brief nonverbal displays affect neuroendocrine levels and risk tolerance. *Psychol Sci* 2010;21(10):1363–1368.

Cherry K. Types of nonverbal communication, n.d. Available at http://psychology.about.com/od/nonverbalcommunication/a/nonverbaltypes.htm. Accessed 18 November 2013.

Ciechanowski PS, Hirsch I B, Katon WJ. Interpersonal predictors of HbA$_{1c}$ in patients with type 1 diabetes. *Diabetes Care* 2002;25(4):731–736.

Cooperrider DL, et al. (Eds). *Lessons from the Field: Applying Appreciative Inquiry.* Bend, OR, Thin Book Publishing, 2001.

Davidson NK, Moreland P. Psychological insulin resistance stems from fear. *Mayo Clinic Living With Diabetes Blog,* 2012. Available at http://www.mayoclinic.com/health/psychological-insulin-resistance/MY01165. Accessed 27 December 2013.

De Jong P, Berg IK. *Interviewing for Solutions.* Belmont, CA, Brooks/Cole, 2008.

Diller JV. *Cultural Diversity.* 3rd ed. Belmont, CA, Brooks/Cole, 2007.

DiMatteo MR. Social support and patient adherence to medical treatment: a meta-analysis. *Psycho Health* 2004;l(23):207–218.

Dingfelder S. Our stories, ourselves. *APA Monitor* 2011;42(1):60.

Dunn SL, Olamijulo GB, et al. The State-Trait Hopelessness Scale: development and testing. *J Nurs Res* 2014;36(4):552–570.

Dweck C. *Mindset: The New Psychology of Success.* New York, NY, Ballantine Books, 2007.

Enzlin P, Rosen R, Wiegel M, Brown J, Wessells H, Gatcomb P, Rutledge B, Chan KL, Cleary PA, DCCT/EDIC Research Group. Sexual dysfunction in women with type 1 diabetes: long-term findings from the DCCT/ EDIC study cohort. *Diabetes Care* 2009;32(5):780–785.

Faber A, Mazlish E. *How to Talk So Teens Will Listen & Listen So Teens Will Talk.* New York, NY, HarperCollins Publishers, 2010.

Fiscella K, Meldrum S, Franks P, Shields CG, Duberstein P, McDaniel SH, Epstein RM. Patient trust: is it related to patient-centered behavior of primary care physicians? *Med Care* 2004;42(11):1049–1055.

Fisher L, Skaff MM, Mullan JT, Arean P, Mohr D, Hasharani U, Glasgow R, Laurencin G. Clinical depression versus distress among patients with type 2 diabetes. *Diabetes Care* 2007;30:542–548.

Fisher L, Gonzalez JS, Polonsky WH. The confusing tale of depression and distress in patients with diabetes: a call for greater clarity and precision. *Diabet Med* 8 March 2014. doi: 10.1111/dme.12428.

Ford D. *The Dark Side of the Light Chasers*. New York, NY, Riverhead Books, 2010.

Freedman J, Combs G. *Narrative Therapy*. New York, NY, W.W. Norton & Company, 1996.

Freire MD, Alves C. Therapeutic Chinese exercises (Qigong) in the treatment of type 2 diabetes mellitus: a systematic review. *Diabetes Metab Syndr* 2013;7(1):56–59.

Gallant M. Help or hindrance? How family and friends influence chronic illness self-management among older adults (report). *Res Aging* 2007;29(5): 375-409.

Gignon M, Idris H, Manaouil C, Ganry O. The waiting room: vector for health education? the general practitioner's point of view. *BMC Res Notes* 2012;18(5):511–516.

Gimenez MC, Hessels M, van de Werken M, de Vries B, Beersma DG, Gordijn MC. Effects of artificial dawn on subjective ratings of sleep inertia and dim light melatonin onset. *Chronobiol Int* 2010;27(6):1219–1241.

Giugliano F, Maiorino MI, Di Palo C, Autorino R, De Sio M, Giugliano D, Esposito K. Women's sexual health: adherence to Mediterranean diet and sexual function in women with type 2 diabetes. *J Sex Med* 2010;7(5):1883–1890.

Goetzke K. How long does it take an action to become a habit; 21, 28, or 66 days? *Psych Central*, 2010. Available at http://blogs.psychcentral.com/adhd/2010/05/how-long-does-it-take-an-action-to-become-a-habit-21-28-or-66-days. Accessed 7 November 2013.

Goldenberg H, Goldenberg I. *Family Therapy An Overview*. 7th ed. Belmont, CA, Thomson Brooks/Cole, 2008.

Goldstein DE, et al. Tests of glycemia in diabetes. *Diabetes Care* 2004;27(7): 1761–1773.

Goleman D. *Emotional Intelligence: Why It Can Matter More than IQ*. New York, Bantam Books, 1997.

Gottman JM. *The Marriage Clinic*. New York, NY, W.W. Norton & Company, 1999.

Grant A. *Give and Take: A Revolutionary Approach to Success.* New York, NY, Viking, 2013.

Gregoire C. This simple mental trick can slow down time. *Huffington Post 10 July 2013.* Available at http://www.huffingtonpost.com/2013/08/20/slow-down-time_n_3567218.html. Accessed 3 June 2014.

Gualtieri L. Doctors need more eye contact with patients, not computers. Kevinmd.com, 2010. Available at http://www.kevinmd.com/blog/2010/04/doctors-eye-contact-patients-computers.html. Accessed 12 August 2013.

Gupta S. Diabetics carry an extra burden of shame. EverydayHealth.com. 24 April 2014. Available at http://www.everydayhealth.com/sanjay-gupta/diabetics-carry-an-extra-burden-of-shame.aspx. Accessed 22 October 2013.

Harley S. *How to Say Anything to Anyone: A Guide to Building Business Relationships That Really Work.* Austin, TX, Greenleaf Book Group, 2013.

Harvard Mental Health Letter. October, 2011. Available at http://www.health.harvard.edu/newsletters/Harvard_Mental_Health_Letter/2011/October/mind-over-matter. Accessed 27 May 2014.

Health Information Privacy. 2008. Available at http://www.hhs.gov/ocr/privacy/hipaa/faq/health_information_technology/570.html. Accessed 8 April 2014.

Hendrix H. *Getting the Love You Want.* New York, NY, Henry Holt, 2008.

Hindi-Alexander M. Compliance or noncompliance: that is the question! *Am J Health Promotion* 1987;1:5–11.

Hodorowicz M. M.O.T.I.V.A.T.E., don't dictate! 33 easy motivational interviewing and adult learning patient counseling tools for diabetes professionals. Poster presentation, American Association of Diabetes Conference, 2013.

Hofmann SG, Asnaani A, Vonk IJJ, Sawyer AT, Fang A. The efficacy of cognitive behavioral therapy: a review of meta-analyses. *Cognit Ther Res* 2012;36(5):427–440.

Hojat M, Louis DZ, Markham FW, Wender, Rabinowitz RC, Gonnella JS. Physicians' empathy and clinical outcomes for diabetic patients. *Acad Med* 2011;86(3):359–364.

Holt RI, Kalra S. A new DAWN: Improving the psychosocial management of diabetes. *Indian J Endocrinol Metab* 2013;17(Suppl. 1):S95–S99.

Horden P (Ed). *Music as Medicine: the History of Music Therapy since Antiquity.* United Kingdom, Ashgate Publishing, 2000, p. 51–68.

Hornbacher M. *Waiting: A Nonbeliever's Higher Power.* Center City, MN, Hazelden, 2011.

Hu J, Wallace DC, McCoy TP, Amirehsani KA. A family-based diabetes intervention for Hispanic adults and their family members. *Diabetes Educ* 18 November 2013 [Epub ahead of print].

Huffington Post: How a (very) little, daily favor can change your life, 2013. Available at http://www.huffingtonpost.com/2013/09/03/five-minute-favor-adam-rifkin_n_3805090.html. Accessed 19 November 2013.

Jantos M, Kiat H. Prayer as medicine: how much have we learned? *Med J Aust* 2007;186(10):S51–S53.

Johnson SM, Wittenborn AK. New research findings on emotionally focused therapy: introduction to special section. *J Marital Fam Ther* 2012;38(Suppl. 1): 18–22.

Jung C. *Psychology and Religion: West and East (The Collected Works of C. G. Jung, Volume 11).* Princeton, NJ, Princeton University Press, 1975.

Kaplan A. *Jewish Meditation: A Practical Guide.* New York, NY, Schocken Books, 1995.

Katz N. Personal communication, 2 December 2013.

Kim H, Schimmack U, Shigehiro O. Cultural differences in self- and other-evaluations and well-being: a study of European and Asian Canadians. *J Pers Soc Psychol* 2012;102(4):856–873.

Kushnir T, Jushnir A, Sarel A, Cohen AH. Exploring physician perceptions of the impact of emotions on behaviour during interactions with patients. *Fam Pract* 2011;28(1):75–81.

Lally P, van Jaarsveld CH, Potts HW, Wardle J. How are habits formed: modelling habit formation in the real world. *Eur J Soc Psychol* 2010;40(6): 998–1009.

Lang EV, Hatsiopoulou O, Koch T, Berbaum K, Lutgendorf S, Kettenmann E, Logan H, Kaptchuk TJ. Can words hurt? Patient-provider interactions during invasive procedures. *Pain* 2005;114(1-2):303–309.

Linzer M, Levine R, Meltzer D, Poplau S, Warde C, West CP. 10 bold steps to prevent burnout in general internal medicine. *J Gen Intern Med* 2014;29(1):18–20.

Leslie CA, Satin-Rapaport W, Matheson D, Stone R, Enfield G. Psychological insulin resistance: a missed diagnosis? *Diabetes Spectr* 1994;7(1):52–57.

LeVan A. Seeing is believing: the power of visualization. *Psychology Today* 2009 Dec 3. Available at http://www.psychologytoday.com/blog/flourish/200912/seeing-is-believing-the-power-visualization. Accessed 23 May 2014.

Lovato N, Lack L. The effects of napping on cognitive functioning. *Prog Brain Res* 2010;185:155–166.

Lowes L, Lyne P. Chronic sorrow in parents of children with newly diagnosed diabetes: a review of the literature and discussion of the implications for nursing practice. *J Adv Nurs* 2000;32(1):41–48.

Lum T. Health-wealth association among older Americans: racial and ethnic differences. *Social Work Res* 2004;28(2):105–116.

Mandel SE, et al. Effects of music therapy and music-assisted relaxation and imagery on health-related outcomes in diabetes education: A feasibility study. *Diabetes Educ* 2013;39(4):568–581.

Marrero DG, Anderson R, Funnell MM, Maryniuk MD. *1,000 Years of Diabetes Wisdom.* Alexandria, VA, American Diabetes Association, 2008.

Mayo Clinic Staff. Forgiveness: letting go of grudges and bitterness. *Mayo Clinic Adult Health*, 23 November 2011. Available at http://www.mayoclinic.com/health/forgiveness/MH00131. Accessed 29 December 2013.

McCoy RG, Van Houten HK, Ziegenfuss JY, Shah ND, Wermers RA, Smith SA. Self-report of hypoglycemia and health-related quality of life in patients with type 1 and type 2 diabetes. *Endocr Pract* 2013;19(5):792–799.

McCullough ME, Kilpatrick SD, Emmons RA, Larson DB. Is gratitude a moral affect? *Psychol Bull* 2001;127(2):249–266.

McGonigal K. Exercise and the immune system: a stress lesson. The science of willpower. 22 October 2009. Available at http://www.psychologytoday.com/blog/the-science-willpower/200910/exercise-and-the-immune-system-stress-lesson. Accessed 13 November 2013.

McGonigal K. *The Willpower Instinct: How Self-Control Works, Why It Matters, and What You Can Do to Get More of It.* New York, NY, Avery, 2011.

McGuire BE, Morrison TG, Hermanns N, Skovlund S, Eldrup E, Gagliardino J, Kokoszka A, Matthews D, Pibernik-Okanović M, Rodríguez-Saldaña J, de Wit M, Snoek FJ. Short-form measures of diabetes-related emotional distress: the Problem Areas in Diabetes Scale (PAID)-5 and PAID-1. *Diabetologia* 2010; 53(1):66–69.

Mehl MR, Vazire S, Ramirez-Esparza N, Slatcher RB, Pennebaker JW. Are women really more talkative than men? *Science* 2007;317(5834):82.

Mikesell L. Medicinal relationships: caring conversation. *Med Educ* 2013;47(5):443–452.

Neff K: *Self-Compassion: Stop Beating Yourself up and Leave Insecurity Behind.* New York, William Morrow, 2011.

Nisselle P. Is self-disclosure a boundary violation? *J Gen Intern Med* 2004;19(9):984.

Norcross JC (Ed). *Psychotherapy Relationships that Work: Therapist Contributions and Responsiveness to Patients.* London, U.K., Oxford University Press, 2002.

Novo Nordisk A/S: DAWN2™ study results, 2013. Available at http://www.dawnstudy.com/dawn2/dawn-2-study-results.asp. Accessed 7 April 2014.

Ofri D. Danielle Ofri on doctors and emotions. Maiken Scott's The Pulse radio program. 5 December 2013b. Available at http://www.newsworks.org/index.php/local/the-pulse/62062-danielle-ofri-. Accessed 31 December 2013.

Ofri D. *What Doctors Feel: How Emotions Affect the Practice of Medicine.* Boston, MA, Beacon Press, 2013a.

Oulasvirta A, Rattenbury T, Ma L, Raita E. Habits make smartphone use more pervasive. *Personal and Ubiquitous Computing* 2012;16(1):105–114.

Palladino DK, Helgeson VS. Friends or foes? A review of peer influence on self-care and glycemic control in adolescents with type 1 diabetes. *J Pediatr Psychol* 2012;37(5):591–603.

Pan A, Lucas M, Sun Q, van Dam RM, Franco OH, Manson JE, Willett WC, Ascherio A, Hu FB. Bidirectional association between depression and type 2 diabetes in women. *Arch Intern Med* 2010;170(21):1884–1891.

Parker-Pope T. Talking to patients after a medical mistake. *Personal and Ubiquitous Computing* 2010;16(1):105–114. Available at http://www.well.blogs.nytimes.com/2010/08/19/talking-to-patients-after-a-medical-mistake/?_r=0. Accessed 9 December 2013.

Peluso P, et al. Relationship education impact reports. PAIRS Foundation, September 2011, for the U.S. Department of Health and Human Services, Administration for Children and Families. Paul Peluso, Ph.D., Principal Investigator, September 2011.

Penson RT, Partridge RA, Rudd P, Seiden MV, Nelson JE, Chabner BA, Lynch TJ Jr. Laughter: the best medicine? *The Oncologist* 2005;10(8):651–660.

Pereira M, Berg-Cross L, Almeida P, Machado J. Impact of family environment and support on adherence, metabolic control, and quality of life in adolescents with diabetes. *Int J Behav Med* 2008;15:187–193.

Peterson CK. Anger and testosterone: evidence that situationally-induced anger relates to situationally-induced testosterone. *Emotion* 2012;12(5):899–902.

Peyrot M, Rubin RR, Lauritzen T, Snoek FJ, Matthews DR, Skovlund SE. Psychosocial problems and barriers to improved diabetes management: results of the cross-national Diabetes Attitudes, Wishes, and Needs study. *Diabet Med* 2005;22:1379–1385.

Pillay S. The art of hugging. *Psychology Today,* 2010. Available at http://www.psychologytoday.com/blog/debunking-myths-the-mind/201007/the-art-hugging. Accessed 11 December 2013.

Polonsky WH. *Diabetes Burnout: What to do When You Can't Take It Anymore.* Alexandria, VA, American Diabetes Association, 1999.

Polonsky WH. Emotional and quality-of-life aspects of diabetes management. *Curr Diab Rep* 2002;2(2):153–159.

Potera C. Words can hurt. *Am J Nurs* 2010;110(12):19.

Powers MA. Diabetes BASICS: education, innovation, revolution. *Diabetes Spectr* 2006;19(2):90–98.

Rapaport W. *When Diabetes Hits Home: The Whole Family's Guide to Emotional Health.* Alexandria, VA, American Diabetes Association, 1989.

Rapaport W. Humor, n.d. Available at http://www.diabetespsyche-drwendy.com/topics/laugh.html. Accessed 2 December 2013.

Ratey J. *Spark: The Revolutionary New Science of Exercise and the Brain.* New York, Little, Brown and Co., 2008.

Roberson CM. Nonverbal communication. *The Alabama Nurse.* September–October 2010.

Rodriguez K. Personal communication. 8 October 2013.

Rogers CR: *A Way of Being.* New York, NY, Houghton Mifflin Company, 1980.

Rolland JS. *Families, Illness, and Disability.* New York, NY, Basic Books, 1994.

Roszler J. Senior pumpers: some seniors may benefit from pump therapy even more than young people do. *Diabetes Forecast* 2002;55(4):37–40.

Roszler J, Polonsky WH, Edelman SV. *The Secrets of Living and Loving with Diabetes*. Chicago, IL, Surrey Books, 2004.

Roszler J, Rice D. *Sex and Diabetes: For Him and For Her*. Alexandria, VA, American Diabetes Association, 2007.

Rubin BM. Many Americans skip vacation time in rough economy, study shows. *Chicago Tribune*, 2012. Available at http://articles.chicagotribune. com/2012-09-03/news/ct-met-no-vacation-20120903_1_vacation-time-free-time-kelton-research. Accessed 13 December 2013.

Sánchez-Villegas A, Delgado-Rodríguez M, Alonso A, Schlatter J, Lahortiga F, Serra Majem L, Martínez-González MA. Association of the Mediterranean dietary pattern with the incidence of depression: the Seguimiento Universidad de Navarra/University of Navarra follow-up (SUN) cohort. *Arch Gen Psychiatry* 2009;66(10):1090–1098, 2009.

Sánchez-Villegas A, Verberne L, De Irala J, Ruíz-Canela M, Toledo E, et al. Dietary fat intake and the risk of depression: the SUN project. *PLoS ONE* 2011;6(1):e16268. Available at http://www.eurekalert.org/pub_releases/2011-01/plos-epc012411.php. Accessed 19 May 2013.

Schnarch D. *Intimacy & Desire*. New York, NY, Beaufort Books, 2009.

Schwartz C, Meisenhelder JB, Ma Y, Reed G. Altruistic social interest behaviors are associated with better mental health. *Psychosom Med* 2003;65(5):778–785.

Seear KH, Vella-Brodrick DA. Efficacy of positive psychology interventions to increase well-being: examining the role of dispositional mindfulness. *Social Indicators Research* 2013;114(3):1125–1141.

Skovlund SE, Peyrot M, on behalf of the DAWN International Advisory Panel. The Diabetes Attitudes, Wishes, and Needs (DAWN) program: a new approach to improving outcomes of diabetes care. *Diabetes Spectrum* 2005;18:136–142.

Smyth JM, Stone AA, Hurewitz A, Kaell A. Effects of writing about stressful experiences on symptom reduction in patients with asthma or rheumatoid arthritis: a randomized trial. *JAMA* 1999;281(14):1304–1309.

Tassi P, Muzet A. Sleep inertia. *Sleep Med Rev* 2000;4(4):341–353.

Tedmed. Dr. Peter Attia, Obesity, 2013. Available at https://www.ted.com/talks/peter_attia_what_if_we_re_wrong_about_diabetes. Accessed 27 May 2014.

Tierney J. A serving of gratitude may save the day. *New York Times* 2011:D1.

Toll BA, Martino S, Latimer A, Salovey P, O'Malley S, Carlin-Menter S, Hopkins J, Wu R, Celestino P, Cummings KM. Randomized trial: quitline specialist training in gain-framed vs standard-care messages for smoking cessation. *J Natl Cancer Inst* 2010;102(2):96–106.

Torosian MH, Biddle VR. Spirituality and healing. *Semin Oncol* 2005;32(2): 232–236.

Vasquez NA, Buehler R. Seeing future success: does imagery perspective influence achievement motivation? *Pers Soc Psychol Bull* 2007;33:1392–1405.

Verschuren, JE, Enzlin P, Dijkstra PU, Geertzen JH, Dekker R. Chronic disease and sexuality: a generic conceptual framework. *J Sex Research* 2010;47:153–170.

Weng HC. Does the physicians' emotional intelligence matter? Impacts of the physician's emotional intelligence on the trust, patient-physician relationship, and satisfaction. *Health Care Manag Rev* 2008;33(4):280–288.

White M. *Maps of Narrative Practice.* New York, NY, W.W. Norton & Company, 2007.

Wise J. How real life change happens, 2013. Available at http://www.psychologytoday.com/blog/extreme-fear/201303/how-real-life-change-happens. Accessed 25 June 2013.

Wood AM, Froh JJ, Geraghty AW. Gratitude and well-being: a review and theoretical integration. *Clin Psychol Rev* 2010;30(7):890–905.

Yalom ID. *The Theory and Practice of Group Psychotherapy.* 5th ed. New York, NY, Basic Books, 2005.

Zrebiec J. Tips for running a successful group. *Diabetes Spectrum* 2003; 16:108–110.

Zrebiec J, Musen G. Emotions & blood-sugar levels: how diabetes can affect your mood. Joslin Diabetes Blog, 2011. Available at http://blog.joslin.org/2011/02/emotions-blood-sugar-levels-how-diabetes-can-affect-your-mood. Accessed 25 December 2013.

Zwolinski R, Zwolinski CR. Therapy tools: role playing. *Psych Central,* 2011. Available at http://blogs.psychcentral.com/therapy-soup/2011/01/therapy-tools-role-playing. Accessed 13 November 2013.

Resources

Quizzes

Use the following quizzes to assess your male and female patients for sexual complications (Roszler, 2007). Positive responses indicate issues that may require attention.

Quiz 1: Have Diabetes-Related Sexual Complications Entered Your Life (for Men)?

1. Have you been experiencing difficulty recently in achieving erections that you and your partner consider adequate for vaginal intercourse?
    ☐ Yes   ☐ No

2. Do you have difficulty performing intercourse in more than half of your attempts?
    ☐ Yes   ☐ No

3. Does this problem with erection difficulty occur when you are with a partner?
    ☐ Yes   ☐ No

4. Does this problem with erection difficulty occur when you are alone?
    ☐ Yes   ☐ No

5. How often have you been experiencing difficulty in achieving erections?   Never   Sometimes   Most times   Always

6. Does it take longer to achieve an erection than in the past?
    ☐ Yes   ☐ No

7. Has it become more difficult to have intercourse in certain positions?
    ☐ Yes   ☐ No

8. Have you ever been told that you have some form of cardiovascular disease or heart disease?
    ☐ Yes   ☐ No

9. Have you ever been told that you have an elevated cholesterol level?
    ☐ Yes   ☐ No

10. Has your desire for intercourse changed?

☐ Yes   ☐ No

11. Has your partner's desire for intercourse changed?

☐ Yes   ☐ No

12. Is your blood glucose under control?

☐ Yes   ☐ No

13. Do you know your average blood glucose level (A1C)?

☐ Yes   ☐ No

14. Have you ever checked your blood sugar level before or after sexual intercourse?

☐ Yes   ☐ No

15. If yes, do you experience hypoglycemia (low blood glucose) with this activity?

☐ Yes   ☐ No

16. Do you feel that diabetes is a cause of your sexual problem?

☐ Yes   ☐ No

17. Has your sexual problem interfered with your relationship with your partner?

☐ Yes   ☐ No

18. Has your sexual problem interfered with your job?

☐ Yes   ☐ No

19. Has your sexual problem interfered with your family?

☐ Yes   ☐ No

20. Are you feeling depressed over this problem?

☐ Yes   ☐ No

Quiz 2: Have Diabetes-Related Sexual Complications Entered Your Life (for Women)?

1. Describe your desire for intercourse.
   Poor   Fair   Strong   Very strong

2. Describe your partner's desire for intercourse.
   Poor   Fair   Strong   Very strong

3. Are you able to reach orgasm with intercourse?
   Never   Sometimes   Most times   Always

4. Are you able to reach orgasm when you are alone?
   Never   Sometimes   Most times   Always

5. Do you have a decreased amount of vaginal lubrication?
   Never   Sometimes   Most times   Always

6. Is your blood glucose under control?
   Never   Sometimes   Most times   Always

7. Do you know your average blood glucose level (low blood glucose)?
   ☐ Yes ☐ No

8. Have you checked your blood glucose before or after sexual intercourse?   ☐ Yes ☐ No

9. If yes, do you experience hypoglycemia (low blood glucose) with this activity?   ☐ Yes ☐ No

10. Do you have frequent vaginal or bladder infections?
    ☐ Yes ☐ No

11. Is intercourse painful?
    ☐ Yes ☐ No

12. Has your sexual problem interfered with your relationship with your partner?   ☐ Yes ☐ No

13. Has your sexual problem interfered with your job?
    ☐ Yes ☐ No

14. Has your sexual problem interfered with your family?
    ☐ Yes ☐ No

15. Are you feeling very depressed over this problem?
    ☐ Yes ☐ No

Validated Tools

The following tools have been validated for assessing the presence of diabetes-related distress (McGuire, 2010).

PAID Questionnaire (Joslin Diabetes Center, 1999).

Available at http://dawnstudy.com/News_and_activities/Documents/ PAID_problem_areas_in_diabetes_questionnaire.pdf

PAID–1

Ask question 12 from the PAID Questionnaire.

PAID–5

Ask questions 3, 6, 12, 16, and 19 from the PAID Questionnaire.

Websites

AADE
American Association of Diabetes Educators
http://www.diabeteseducator.org

AAMFT
American Association for Marriage and Family Therapy
http://www.aamft.org/iMIS15/AAMFT

ADA
American Diabetes Association
http://www.diabetes.org

APA
American Psychological Association
http://www.apa.org

Dulwich Centre
A gateway to information about narrative therapy and collective narrative practice.
http://www.dulwichcentre.com.au

ICEEFT
The International Centre for Excellence in Emotionally Focused Therapy
http://iceeft.com

Integrated Diabetes Services
A source for therapists who understand diabetes-related issues and offer phone or video messaging sessions; all of the clinicians associated with this website have diabetes.
http://www.integrateddiabetes.com

NASW
National Association of Social Workers
http://socialworkers.org

NDEP
National Diabetes Education Program
Video: "Partnering with Your Diabetes Care Team"
http://ndep.nih.gov/resources/diabetes-healthsense/index.aspx

Positive Psychology Center
University of Pennsylvania
http://www.ppc.sas.upenn.edu

Index

A

Accusatory language, 50
Acknowledgment, 32, 35
Active listening, 33–34
Adolescents, 127–129
Affirmation, 35, 49, 54, 94
Agenda setting, 13
Altruism, celebration of, 94–95
Anger, 76–77
Anticipation, 48
Anxiety, 77–78
Appreciation, 49–50
Appreciations, 137–138
Approach-avoidance behavior, 40
Assertive language, 50–51
Attachment histories, 40
Attachment issues, 40–41
Attia, Peter, 84
Authority figures, 95–96

B

Behavioral health referrals, 43–45
Behavioral health screening, 53
Behaviors, at home, 136
Beliefs, 16. See also spirituality

Blood glucose drop, 77
Blood glucose monitoring,
        patient worksheets on, 23
Body language, 106–107, 119–120
Boundaries, 51
Breathing, 8
Brewer, Judson, 82
Button pushing, 41–43

C

"Call it a day," 132
Calming tools, 8–9. See also Stop, Drop,
        and Roll (SDR)
Challenging patients, 39–40, 41–45
Challenging situations, 47–48. See also
        emotional sessions
Circular relationships, 2
Cognitive restructuring, 52
Collaboration
        communication and, 52–53
        relationship building and, 32, 37
Collaborative conversation, 52–53
Communication, 37–38
        emotional sessions and, 50, 52–53, 53–55
        externalizing conversations, 55–56

home-life and, 137–139
mental health and, 44–45
nonverbal, 111–112
patient connections and, 33–34, 37–38
questions and, 65, 69, 72, 73–74
in the workplace, 109–111
See also listening
Commuting, 7
Compassion, 34
Confrontation
empathic, 54
with patient families, 120
in the workplace, 112–113
Connecting with patients. *See* patient
connections
Connection enhancement, 137–139
Coping strategies, 96
Criticism, 50
Cuddy, Amy, 106
Cultural beliefs, 38
Cultural sensitivity, 121

D
Day review, 133–134
Deep breathing, 8
Defensiveness, 78
Deficit-focused conversation, 69
Denial, 79
Depression, 80, 85
Diabetes Attitudes, Wishes, and
Needs (DAWN) study, 43–44
Diabetes police, 26
Diabetes Progress Scale, 27, 28–29
Diabetes-related distress, 80
Diet
for care providers, 6–7
for patients, 21
Directness, 110–111
Disclaimers, 110
Disruptions, in group sessions, 97–98

E
Education, 13, 53. *See also* patient education
Embarrassment, 80–81
Emotional literacy, 75
Emotional sessions

anticipation and, 48–49
collaboration and, 52–53, 58–60
communication and, 50, 52–55
pointing out patient upsets in, 61–62
positive care provider response, 49–50,
51–52, 54, 56–58, 62, 64, 66, 69–71, 72
See also moods
Emotional state: of patients, 1–2.
See also Emotional sessions; moods
Emotions, common for patients, 76–88
Empathic confrontation, 54
Empathic language, 50–51
Empathy, 35–35, 36, 54, 61
Encouragement, 55–56
End-of-life issues, 124–125
Environment, 12
Exceptions, search for, 65–66
Externalizing conversations, 55–56
Extroversion, 107

F
Fear, 81–83
Feeling, 108
"Fighting" fair, in the workplace, 112–113
Fisher, L., 80
Five-minute favors, 114
Forgiveness, 57–58
Frustration, 24, 83, 99
Functional impairment, 80

G
Gifts of Imperfection, The (Brown, 2010), 84
Glucose level checks, 12–13
Goals, 18
Grant, Adam, 109–110
Gratitude, 19, 49–50, 57
Group participation
closing the session, 101–102
dealing with challenges, 97–98
logistics, 102–103
new leadership and, 103–104
positive action in, 93–97
scenarios possible in, 98–101
types of interactions, 90
Guided imagery meditation, 9
Guilt, 83–84, 120–121

H
Harley, Shari, 105–106
Hate, 84–85
Healthy eating, 21
Healthy habits, care provider, 135
Hedges, 110
Hendrix, Harville, 76–77
Hesitations, 110
Home-life, 140
  behaviors and, 136
  communication and, 137–139
  connection enhancement
      and, 137–139
  mindfulness and, 134–135;
      Stop, Drop, and Roll (SDR)
      and, 132–133
Hope, 94
Hopelessness, 85–86
Humor, 57–58
Hurt, 86
Hypoglycemia, 77

I
"I don't know," 126–127
Influence over others, 114–115
Inner voice, 4–6
Instructions, in a group setting, 91–92
Insulin pump use, 99–100
Intimacy issues, 80–81, 123–124
Intimate partnerships, 122–123
Introversion, 107
Intuition, 108

J
Journaling, 58–59
Jung, Carl, 42

K
Katz, Nathan, 124
Kid's behavior, 125–129

L
Language, 50–51, 109–111
LEAP, 95–96, 119
Letter writing, 58–59

Listening, 33–34
Loss, 124–125

M
Marriage, 122–123
McGonigal, K., 88
Meditation, 9
Mental health, 43–44
Micromanagement, 122–123
Mindfulness, 9, 68, 134–135
Minute visualization, 9
Mismanagement accusations, 120
Moods
  impact of diet on, 6–7
  patient connections and, 32
  tools for improved, 8–9
  See also emotional sessions;
      emotional state
Morning preparations, 2–9
Motivation, lack of, 88
Motivational interviewing, 59–60

N
Naming emotions, 61–62
Negative message management, 4–6
Negative responses, care provider, 41
"Next time" guide, 75–88
Nonverbal communication, 111–112

O
Overwhelming emotions, 24

P
Parents, 127–128
Passing feelings, 56
Passover, 38
Patient behavior, improvement of, 38–39.
      See also patient connections
Patient connections
  affirmations and, 35
  empathy and, 34–35
  challenges to, 39–45
  communication and, 33–34, 37–38
  positively reframe and, 36–37
Patient dislike, 39–45
Patient education, 13–27, 53

Patient family interactions, 117–118
  children and, 125–129
  patient input and, 118–119
  social dynamics and, 121–124
Patient feelings, 43–44. *See also* moods
Patient interaction
  and the Diabetes Progress Scale, 27–29
  mood and, 1–2
  with staff, 11–12
  worksheets and, 13–27. *See also* emotional
    sessions; group participation;
    patient connections
Patient moods. *See* moods
Patient referrals, psychology specialist, 43–45
Patient tools of self-expression and, 58–59
Patient worksheets, 13–17
Patient-staff interactions, 11–12
Perception, of care providers, 108–109
Personal awkwardness, 80–81
Personal beliefs, 16
Personal goals, 18
Personal stories, 66–67
Personalizing sessions, 97
Physical activity, 8–9, 22
Physical stances, 106–107
Physicians' models, 2
Positive thinking, 17
Positive verbal attention, 2
Positively reframe, 36–37, 54, 62–63
Prayer, 63
Problem Area in Diabetes Scale (PAID), 80
Problem identification, 55
Professional network, 62
Progress, 27
Provider emotions
  defensiveness, 78
  frustration, 83
  sadness, 87
  See also Stop, Drop, and Roll (SDR)

Q
Quitting time, 131–132

R
Ramadan, 38
Ratey, John, 113

Reflecting, 71–72
Reinforcement, 63–64
Relatives, 120–121. *See also* patient family
    interactions
Repression, 42
Reprioritization, 64
Resentment, 76–77
Respect, for co-workers, 107
Responsiveness, to patient emotions, 61–62,
    66–67, 70–74. *See also* emotional
    sessions
Ritual quitting time, 132
Role-playing, 64, 93
Rule review, in a group setting, 92–93

S
Sadness, 86–87, 100–101
Scaling questions, 65
Self-awareness, 41–43, 108–111
Self-care behaviors, 14
Self-compassion, 66
Self-disclosure, 66
Self-talk, 4–6, 67–68
Sensing, 108
Sex and Diabetes (Roszler, 2007), 123–124
Sexual complication quizzes
Sexual complications, 80–81, 124
"Shadow," 42
Shame, 83–84
Sharing, group, 94
Silence, in group sessions, 97, 100
Skills, learning new, 25
Sleep inertia, 3–4
Social behaviors, successful, 96
Social support, 15, 26, 86, 118–119. *See also*
    patient family interactions
Solution identification, 56
Solution-focused family therapy
    approach, 59, 65
Spirituality, 63, 121–122
Staff, 11–12. *See also* workplace interactions
Staff-patient interactions, 11–12
Starting your day. *See* morning preparations
Stop, Drop, and Roll (SDR), 4–6, 48, 70
  common emotions and, 77–88
  in group sessions, 97–98, 99

home-life and, 132–133
    patient families and, 119
Storytelling, 66–67, 70–71
Strength-based questions, 69–70, 73–74,
    125–126
Strengths-focused conversation, 69–70
Stress, 87–88
Stress management, patient, 20
Support groups, 72
Support value, 15

T

Tag questions, 110
Technology, new, 78
Thankfulness, 19
Therapy, 44
Thinking styles, 108
Thinking, 108
Thought accuracy, 52
Thought-tracking, 52
Time out, 73
Transference, 58, 109

Trust, in care providers, 2
Type 2 Diabetes (T2D), 80, 83–84

V

Vacations, 139
Validation, 49
Verbosity, 110–111
Visualization, 9, 73

W

Wait times, 12–13
Waiting area transformation, 12, 13
Weight gain emotions, 55–56
What went well, 73–74, 129, 133
Workplace interactions
    communication and, 109–112
    confidence and, 106–107
    confrontations and, 112–113
    positive actions for, 114–115
    respecting others and, 107
    self-awareness and, 108–109
Worksheets, patient, 13–27
Worry, 77–78